About the author

Dr Vernon Coleman worked as a GP in the Midlands for ten years. He is now a professional author and broadcaster. He was the UK's first TV agony uncle, has made three TV series based on his bestselling book *Bodypower* and has made a special series of programmes on tranquillizers to accompany *Life Without Tranquillisers*. His weekly medical columns appear in newspapers all over the world. He is the author of over thirty books, including *Mindpower* (Century, 1986). His books have been translated into eleven languages; four have been in the 'bestseller' lists. He is a Fellow of the Royal Society of Medicine.

Also available from Century
Mindpower

Other books by Dr Vernon Coleman include
The Home Pharmacy
Face Values
Guilt
Stress and Your Stomach
A Guide to Child Health
Women's Problems: An A–Z
The Good Medicine Guide
Bodypower
Bodysense
Taking Care of Your Skin
Life Without Tranquillisers
Eczema and Dermatitis
High Blood Pressure
Arthritis
Diabetes
The Story of Medicine

NATURAL PAIN CONTROL

Dr Vernon Coleman

CENTURY ARROW
London Melbourne Auckland Johannesburg

A Century Arrow Book
Published by Arrow Books Limited
62–65 Chandos Place, London WC2N 4NW

An imprint of Century Hutchinson Ltd

London Melbourne Sydney Auckland
Johannesburg and agencies throughout
the world

First published 1986

Printed and bound in Great Britain by
Hunt Barnard Printing Ltd, Aylesbury, Bucks

ISBN 0 09 948400 5

Contents

Introduction

It is impossible to work out how many people suffer from persistent or recurrent pain. But, according to figures prepared by one world expert, well over half the adult population suffer from persistent or recurrent pain. Millions are partly or totally disabled by the pain produced by diseases such as arthritis, backache, migraine and cancer. And the cost in medical expenses, lost working days and industrial compensation must be measured in billions of pounds. The cost to the individual cannot be measured.

Persistent or recurrent pain has a fearful effect upon both the body and the mind. It turns strong individuals into weak, nervous folk. It turns the affable into the irritable; it makes cowards of the brave.

We think of pain as being a useful warning sign, a message designed to tell us that all is not well. But too often pain serves no useful purpose at all. Acute pain may be a life saver but chronic pain is the most fearful of all burdens. It turns the sensible into the desperate. Pain makes people vulnerable and turns cautious citizens into easy targets for quacks and charlatans.

The sufferer from persistent or recurrent pain cannot sleep or rest; his hopes will be built up repeatedly and then quickly dashed; he will often find it difficult to explain to others the extent of his pain and suffering. However bizarre they may seem, he will explore all potential possibilities for relief and understanding, support and sympathy. He will struggle to understand what purpose his pain can serve. He will be depressed and discouraged no matter how often he is given hope and encouragement.

Sadly, patients suffering from persistent or recurrent pain

are not well served by the medical profession. Doctors will usually search for some permanent cure, and when none can be found they will become disheartened, disappointed and frustrated. They feel guilty and inadequate and refer their patients to yet another physician or surgeon. The patient will be passed from surgery to clinic to hospital to surgery, trying drugs and operations but too often getting nowhere.

And yet, despite the failure of the medical profession to offer much in the way of useful advice, the fact is that during the last two decades we have learned an enormous amount about what causes pain and about how pain can best be controlled. We still do not have access to immediate and permanent cures. But we do know how pain can be controlled well enough to enable sufferers to lead normal lives.

The Pain Control Programme outlined in this book is not offered as a miracle remedy. It will not cure patients, nor will it banish pain. But it will show how pain can be controlled. A pain that is allowed to grow unfettered will prove crippling and dangerous. A patient who is constantly fighting pain will retire to his bed, abandon his work, and allow himself to sink into a slough of despair from which escape is nigh on impossible. And the more passive a patient becomes, the more fearful and constricting will his pain become.

My Pain Control Programme will help patients gain control over their pain. It will enable patients who suffer from persistent or recurrent pain of any kind to take charge of their lives once more. It will show patients hope for the future and will enable them to harness their own strength and courage in such a way that they will be able to overcome the fearful handicap of persistent, debilitating pain.

Vernon Coleman
Devon, 1986

PART ONE

The Pain Fact File

What Is Pain?

Everyone knows what pain is, but trying to produce a precise definition is a bit like trying to nail jelly to the ceiling. Just when you think you've got things under control it all slips through your fingers and leaves you clutching handfuls of thin air. Pain is the single most common reason why people seek medical attention. It is the most important reason why people take pills. And yet it cannot be measured objectively, and there is no such thing as a standard pain for a specific disease process. For decades eminent medical men have struggled to find an acceptable definition, and all have failed.

The reason for all this confusion is undoubtedly the fact that pain is neither a readily defined sensation nor a strictly regulated response. Between the original stimulus and the individual's perception of that stimulus a huge number of variables intervene, with the result that identical pain-producing stimuli can not only produce different responses when perceived by different individuals, but can also produce different responses when perceived by the same individual on different occasions.

Like the word 'stress', the word 'pain' is something that everyone understands but no one can define to everyone else's satisfaction.

The body's first and most important response to a painful stimulus is to release a number of potent chemical substances. Normally stored in the body's tissues close to a comprehensive and sophisticated network of special nerve endings, which will eventually carry news about the painful stimulus to the brain and the rest of the body's nervous system, these chemicals stimulate those nerve endings almost immediately.

So, for example, if you are trying to hang a picture in the living room and you hit your thumb with a hammer, the tissues of your thumb will immediately release two sets of chemicals known as kinins and prostaglandins. Both these substances sensitize the body's nerve endings and help ensure that messages are sent to your brain telling you that your thumb has been hurt.

In addition to ensuring that these vital messages are transmitted as soon as possible, the prostaglandins will also help increase the flow of blood to the area of your thumb. This increase in circulation will result in your thumb turning red and beginning to swell. The idea behind this is that the increased blood supply will bring in white blood cells to the area and help kill off any infective organisms which may have got into the tissues through a break in the skin. The swelling caused by the extra blood also means that the thumb is difficult to move and will therefore be rested while it recovers.

Whether you hit yourself with a hammer, stand on a tintack, develop a boil or bang your arm on the door much the same sort of thing happens. In each case the injury or inflammation stimulates the local production of these chemicals, and the chemicals in turn ensure that the body's pain-sensitive nerve endings carry the appropriate messages to the brain.

The pain receptors which are triggered by these chemicals and which pass the news on to the body's nervous system can be subdivided into a number of different categories. There are receptors which carry information about extremes of heat or cold, and there are non-specific receptors which simply carry news of all ill-defined pains. There are even receptors which detect the presence in the body of excess quantities of waste chemicals produced during hectic exercise. Normally these chemicals are removed by the circulating blood, but if the circulation is not powerful enough to remove the wastes as quickly as they are accumulating, special pain receptors will be stimulated.

Once the nerve endings have been triggered then the pain signal travels, partly as an electrical impulse and partly as a chemical message, along the appropriate nerve until it reaches the spinal cord. There the pain signal meets all sorts of other messages coming from other parts of the body and finally makes its way up the spinal cord to the brain.

Now, the whole story of just how pain reaches the brain is something of a mystery. Scientists are still studying the whole subject of pain receptors, kinins and prostaglandins. The extent of our ignorance about these simple mechanisms is quite remarkable. Exactly what happens when the pain receptors have been stimulated and the pain message has started its journey along the nerve pathways is more a question of guesswork than of certainty.

The traditional theory, first made popular by Descartes in 1664, was that when a pain receptor is stimulated the pain message travels straight up to the brain. Descartes believed that it was all remarkably simple and rather like a campanologist tugging on a bell rope to start the church bells ringing.

Known as the 'theory of specificity', this simple concept has been taught in medical schools for just about as long as there have been medical schools. Most of the doctors currently in practice were taught this theory as undergraduates, and the theory is still popular in some teaching establishments today.

It is this three-hundred-year-old theory of specificity which has led many doctors to think of pain in very straightforward terms and helped encourage the conclusion that, since the relationship between cause and effect is so simple, the remedy must also be simple. Those doctors who think that Descartes was right believe that pain can be abolished simply by interfering with the transmission of impulses from pain receptor to brain. In simple terms they argue that pain relief is as easy as cutting bell ropes or telephone wires. If you cut the nerve that carries the pain impulse from the receptor then there should be no perception of pain in the brain.

As a theory this all sounds very plausible, but in practice this hypothesis doesn't stand up very well. There are a number of problems with it.

One major problem is that attempts to interfere with chronic or persistent pain by cutting nerve pathways fail as often as they succeed. Indeed, the pain after surgery may be even worse than the original pain.

To this must be added the fact that pain can continue long after the original stimulus has been removed, and that it can occur spontaneously and may spread to apparently unrelated parts of the body. Moreover, during the last twenty years scientists have accumulated an extraordinary amount of evidence showing that the quality and quantity of pain perceived by an individual patient can be determined by numerous psychological factors. Under some circumstances quite intense stimulations can be prevented from causing any pain at all. Under other circumstances terrible pain can be produced by quite modest stimulations.

By the mid-1960s thoughtful scientists had realized that although there undoubtedly are nervous pathways which carry pain messages from peripheral pain receptors to the brain, those pathways are not simple and it is not possible to predict the type of response likely to be obtained by stimulating a specific receptor.

Then in 1965 a psychologist called Ronald Melzack, at the time an Associate Professor at the Massachusetts Institute of Technology, and Patrick Wall, an anatomist, produced their 'gate control theory' which revolutionized the way doctors thought about pain.

Melzack and Wall argued that only a certain amount of sensory information can be processed by the nervous system at any one moment, and that when too much information tries to get through the limited number of junctions in the spinal cord special cells shut out some of the signals. The theory proposed that there is, in the spinal cord, a special mechanism which acts rather like an ordinary garden gate. The gate can only accept a certain number of messages at any one time, and if too many messages try to get through then the gate effectively shuts and blocks off the flow of further messages from peripheral parts of the body to the brain.

The gate control theory rests upon the fact that messages arrive at the spinal cord in three quite separate ways. First, there are two main types of nerve fibre which detect pain and other sensations and which carry electrical impulses produced by the receptors in the body's muscles and tissues. The thicker of these two types of fibre carry sensations such as touch and pressure while the other, thinner fibres carry pain messages. These two fibres differ in various ways. First, the thinner fibres can regrow if they are damaged whereas the thicker fibres cannot regenerate and tend to diminish in number over the years. The second, and much more important difference is that the thicker fibres carry their nervous impulses much more rapidly than the thinner fibres do.

In addition to these messages travelling up towards the brain there are also likely to be instructions of many different kinds travelling down from the brain towards the muscles and other tissues.

Under normal circumstances the junctions in the spinal cord can carry these three different types of messages quite comfortably. But if too many impulses reach the spinal cord the junction cells just can't cope: they shut down and won't accept any additional messages.

It is this inability of the cells in the spinal cord to cope with the number of messages they are getting that explains why some stimuli produce far more savage pains than other apparently comparable stimuli.

To help me explain just how this works try to imagine that you have carelessly hit your thumb with your hammer and then rubbed your thumb vigorously. Because your skin has been damaged and your receptors have been chemically stimulated all sorts of signals will be sent along the nerves towards your spinal cord. There will be sensations of pressure and touch travelling along the thicker fibres. And there will be pain sensations travelling along the thinner fibres. The nerves transmitting messages from your thumb to your brain will be overloaded with information.

Inevitably, the gate will get blocked and some impulses will be unable to get through. And since it is the non-painful signals of pressure and touch, travelling much more speedily along the thicker fibres, which will get there first, they will tend to block the gateway and prevent many of the pain messages getting through at all.

As I will explain more fully later, our habit of rubbing a sore or damaged part is a natural response designed to stimu-late the sending of simple 'sensation' messages and thereby to block the passage of involuntarily produced pain messages.

That is one way in which the gate control theory explains just how pain impulses can be blocked. There is another way in which much the same sort of thing can happen.

If enough messages are coming down from the brain to the tissues then the gate will be blocked from the opposite direction and, once again, the pain messages won't be able to get through. So, if you're concentrating very hard on what you're doing with your hammer then you may not even notice that you've hurt yourself. It is this aspect of the gate control theory which explains why apparently painful incidents are so often ignored by people who are concentrating on what they are doing.

Of course if the number of impulses travelling along the smaller fibres carrying pain messages greatly exceeds both the number of fast-moving messages travelling along the larger fibres and the number of messages coming down from the brain, the pain message will get through the gate and you'll become aware of the pain.

For the first time in several hundred years Melzack and Wall had produced a theory which helped to explain just about all the strange and previously inexplicable aspects of pain. Their theory explained why different people perceived pain in different ways. And it explained why the same individual can respond to an identical stimulus in different ways according to his surroundings and circumstances. It explained how a footballer can carry on playing even though he has a broken arm. It explained how a soldier can continue to fight even though his foot has been shot off. It explains how a man can pick up his severed arm and walk calmly with it to the nearest hospital.

And as one romantic scientist pointed out, it explains how two young lovers can stand out in the freezing cold and not notice that they're getting frostbitten.

The development of the gate control theory didn't just revolutionize the way that doctors think about pain, however; it also helped many people begin to look for new ways of dealing with pain. After all, if the perception of pain can be regulated by other impulses either coming from the skin and tissues or coming from the brain then it must be possible to use those other regulatory mechanisms to help control pain. The gate control theory had helped to explain why pain seemed such an unpredictable force. It also helped open up the way for many other research workers to start examining the whole pain phenomenon far more closely.

The Values and Mysteries of Pain

The patient suffering from chronic backache, persistent arthritis or recurrent migraine attacks may find it difficult to believe, but pain is essential. It helps to protect us in several important ways.

First, pain often helps us to avoid serious injury. If you pick up a red-hot pan that has been left on the stove for too long then the burning pain you feel will ensure that you let go very quickly. If you hadn't felt the pain you would have sustained far more serious burns. If you sit down on a drawing pin then the pain that you feel will ensure that you stand up again pretty quickly.

Second, pain helps us to learn what dangerous situations we should try to avoid and it teaches us to be careful when handling potentially dangerous objects. When you've smashed your thumb a few times with a hammer you'll learn to respect the hammer and use it with more caution. When you've burnt your feet by jumping into a bathtub of boiling water you'll learn to put a little cold water in before you leap into the bath.

Third, pain makes us rest parts of our body which might otherwise be damaged even more by continuous strain and pressure. If you twist your knee running for a bus then the knee will become painful and you'll want to keep off it for a few days. You'll walk with a stick or a crutch and you'll take care not to do any running until the joint has had time to recover.

And finally, pain tells us when we need help. If you have a persistent abdominal pain or a recurrent pain in or around one of your teeth then you will, if you're sensible, call for a doctor or a dentist. Moreover, when you ask for professional advice the expert you see will be able to use the information that you can give him about your pain to help him decide exactly what is wrong and what needs doing. If you have a pain in your foot you're unlikely to need an ear, nose and throat surgeon. If you have a pain in your ear you're unlikely to need a gynaecologist.

There is a rare medical condition in which patients are simply not able to feel pain sensations. And, although such a condition may sound appealing to the chronic pain sufferer, these unfortunate individuals live short and unhappy lives. They burn themselves repeatedly by picking up hot objects or by getting into bath water that is scalding. They stand too near to open fires and set fire to their flesh without realizing what is happening. They walk with broken bones and damage their joints and limbs. They bite their tongues repeatedly when chewing food. And they frequently cut themselves badly when handling knives or saws. If you don't feel pain you don't move your hand away when the bread knife starts to cut into your flesh – you just press harder.

One of the best-documented stories to illustrate the value of pain involves a young Canadian girl who felt no pain at all whatever stimulation was applied to her body. Under laboratory conditions she did not respond to electric shocks, to hot water nor even to having a stick pushed up high into her nostrils. She was totally immune to pain, however terrible. No torture could hurt her.

Because of her inability to feel pain, however, she needed constant medical attention. Her major problem was that she acquired a number of joint disorders. Normally, when we go to bed at night we move about constantly in our sleep in order to ensure that the pressure on our joints and tissues is never allowed to build up to too high a level. It is pain that ensures that we move. When we are standing we constantly and automatically shift our weight from one foot to the other in order to protect our hip, knee and ankle joints. Again it is pain that ensures that we make these minor and automatic but important changes.

However, because her body could feel no pain the young Canadian girl did not move her joints when she slept, stood or sat. And the result was that she acquired a huge number of damaging joint problems. She spent a good part of her later life in hospital but there was nothing that the doctors could do to help her, and she died at the age of twenty-nine of a massive infection that had started in one of those damaged joints. Her inability to feel pain had killed her.

Having now established the value of pain, there are three specific and exceptional aspects of pain which need to be described in more detail: the fact that pain doesn't always tell the truth and isn't always what it seems to be, and that sometimes we feel pain in areas of our bodies far removed from the illness or abnormality that is causing the pain (this is a sometimes confusing phenomenon known as referred pain); the fact that it is often possible for us to endure injury without feeling pain; and, perhaps most important of all, the fact that it is possible to feel pain without there being any injury.

Referred pain

If you have your eyes closed and someone sticks a pin in your thumb then you'll know that the pin has been stuck into your thumb. You'll be able to locate the site of the injury and the pain quite accurately. If someone standing behind you pinches your left earlobe then you'll know instantly exactly where it is that they've pinched you.

The ability to locate a pain accurately only works when it is the skin that has been injured. Pain that occurs inside your body can be very misleading and can relate to problems quite a long way away.

There are one or two reasons why this can occur, but the best way to explain what happens is probably to offer a few examples.

Imagine, for example, that you have just banged the inside of your elbow – it's the area most of us know rather affectionately as our 'funny bone'. Although it is the inside of your elbow that has been banged you will feel pain in your hand and, in particular, in the little finger of that hand.

The explanation is very simple. The nerve that supplies that part of your hand, and which normally carries the pain messages from your little finger to your brain, travels up your arm and at that point, just inside your elbow, runs over the surface of the bone. When you bang your funny bone you compress the nerve and stimulate it to send messages up to your brain. The normal pain pathway that I described at the start of this part of the book has been short-circuited.

Much the same sort of thing can happen if you have a disc lesion low down in your spine. If a disc 'slips' and presses on one of the nerves in your spinal cord which normally carries pain messages from your leg or foot then you'll think you can feel pain coming from your leg or foot. There won't be anything wrong with your leg or foot, of course; the pain will be quite misleading and inappropriate. But it will be a very real pain nevertheless, and almost indistinguishable from the sort of pain you would feel if you did injure your leg or foot.

That sort of referred pain is fairly common and fairly easy to explain. But the majority of referred pains are far more complicated than these and result from changes which take place when we are still developing in our mother's womb.

Consider, for example, one of the commonest of all important abdominal pains: appendicitis. The appendix is a small intestinal cul-de-sac that has no real function but is an evolutionary left-over. It lies deep down in the abdomen and can usually be found on the right-hand side, tucked into the pelvis. Problems develop with the appendix because occasionally small bits of undigested food get stuck in it, and produce infection and inflammation.

Because of its position in the abdomen you would imagine that when the appendix becomes inflamed the pain it produces would also be fairly low down on the right-hand side of the abdomen. But it isn't. To start with the pain of appendicitis develops in the upper abdomen, around or even just above the navel.

The explanation for this bizarre state of affairs is that when we are still developing as embryos, our intestines start as a straight tube, with the appendix situated right in the middle of the abdomen and getting its nerve supply from nerves which also supply the skin and abdominal wall around and just above the navel. It isn't until much later on in our embryonic development that our intestines grow so long that they have to curl up in coils in order to fit into the abdomen.

To start with, therefore, appendicitis produces a pain that seems to come from the area around the navel. It is only as the appendicitis develops and the inflammation spreads that the pain seems to move down into the right-hand side of the lower abdomen. The pain moves because as the inflammation spreads it begins to affect the skin of the abdomen and irritate the nerves which supply the skin directly above it. At this point, several hours after the pain has begun, the pain will accurately pinpoint the site of the trouble.

Two of the other most commonly experienced referred pains are angina (or heart pain) and toothache.

Let's take angina first. Most people imagine that heart pain should be felt on the left-hand side of the chest, where the heart is classically thought to be situated. But it isn't. Classically, a patient suffering from angina will complain of a tight pain across both sides of his chest and of a pain that also goes down his left arm. Once again the explanation for this apparently peculiar phenomenon is quite simple. When we develop as an embryo our heart starts out in the middle of our body. It gets its initial nerve supply from both the right and the left sides of the chest. As the heart develops, the left side grows much larger than the right, since it is the left side which will ultimately have the major responsibility for pumping blood around the body. (The right side of the heart has the smaller but none the less important responsibility for pumping blood back into the lungs for oxygenation). Since it is growing larger than the right side, the left side of the heart needs more nerves, and it gets its extra nerve supplies from the same sources as the left arm.

Finally, consider toothache, another common pain problem that is often very misleading. Patients are for ever turning up at their doctors' consulting rooms complaining of earache when in fact they have a bad tooth that needs attention. And at the dentist, patients will often complain of a pain in one tooth when in fact the pain is being produced by a problem in an entirely different tooth.

Once again all this is quite easily explained. The nerve

supplies to our teeth are developed long before our mouths have been properly formed, and the resulting confusion is hardly surprising. Only if an infection leaks out of a tooth and affects the gums will the pain be felt in precisely the right place. As with any pain, once the superficial tissues have been involved then the source of the pain will be much easier to identify and locate accurately.

Injury without pain

Most of us think of pain as being usually associated with some sort of physical injury. The pain may not always be felt in precisely the right spot. But we believe that if there is an injury then there must nearly always be a pain. And, even more important, we assume that the amount of pain we feel will depend upon the extent of the injury.

Sometimes this assumption is justified. If you hit your thumb with a hammer, but only hit it lightly, then you'll only feel a modest amount of pain. But if you give your thumb a full-blooded whack with a hammer then you'll feel a pretty terrible pain. The harder you hit it the more pain you'll get and the more it will hurt. If you catch your head a glancing blow on a low beam then you'll suffer a slight pain. If you bang your head very hard on a low beam then you'll suffer a much worse pain.

But often this basic assumption that the amount of pain an individual feels must be in direct proportion to the size of the injury he has sustained cannot be justified in practice. There are many times when individuals can experience quite serious injuries without feeling very much pain. So, for example, something like six out of every ten soldiers who are severely wounded in battle will not complain of any pain, while two out of every ten patients who undergo major surgery don't complain of any pain afterwards either. In 1982 three researchers in America found that over a third of all the people who arrived at the emergency clinic of a large hospital, and who had a variety of serious injuries, including major cuts, fractured bones and even amputated fingers, reported that they didn't feel any pain for a long time after their injury.

Perhaps most startling of all are the authenticated stories told by anthropologists who have reported watching native ceremonies in which perfectly sane and sensible people sustain quite horrendous injuries, apparently without feeling pain.

So, for example, every year villagers in a certain part of rural India elect a young man to be king for a day. The election is an important one in village life, for the people believe that the king's blessing will ensure that the village will enjoy good crops and good health for the rest of the year.

As an absolutely vital part of the ceremony large hooks are pushed into the flesh of the elected king's back and the man is then hoisted high into the air so that he dangles above the villagers, held in the sky like a joint of beef at the butcher's. You would imagine that the king would be in agony. But he isn't. He blesses the village with happiness and joy on his face.

A similar sort of thing happens among North American Indians in their Sun Dance ceremony. Incisions are made in the chests of young men and skewers are then pushed through the incisions. As in India, the young men are then hoisted into the air by the skewers through their skin. In this ceremony however the young men are expected to thrash around until they tear themselves free. To do this they have literally to tear the flesh from their chests.

A third example comes from East Africa where both men and women undergo an operation called trepanation. The patients are not anaesthetized while their scalps are removed and large areas of skull are exposed. A local 'doctor' then scrapes the skull as the man or woman sits calmly holding a pan under his or her chin to catch the dripping blood.

These are all slightly bizarre examples of ways in which the human body can be damaged without there being any pain. And later in this book I will explain just why these injuries can be sustained without the people involved feeling pain. But I don't want to leave this short section on 'injury without pain' without pointing out that, although our bodies are very good at producing pain to tell us of external injuries we have sustained, they are not good at telling us of problems that may be developing unseen, deep inside our bodies.

So, although our bodies are extremely good at responding to external injury by producing pain, and although pain provides us with an excellent 'early warning' that can protect us from further physical damage, we can develop huge and inoperable cancers without feeling any pain; we can develop dangerous heart disease without being aware that anything is wrong and we can suffer from malfunctioning livers, brains, kidneys and lungs without receiving any indication from our pain receptors that there is anything wrong.

Pain can often provide a useful warning and it is a vital protective mechanism, but it cannot be depended upon to provide us with information about developing disease.

Pain without injury

The more we examine the relationship between injury and illness on the one hand and pain on the other hand, the clearer it becomes that there is not always a direct link between the two. And just as it is perfectly possible for a serious illness to develop without there being any pain, or for an individual to sustain serious injury apparently without suffering any pain, so it is also possible for individuals to suffer pain without there being any observable injury, or to suffer pain that is far greater than any existing injury might explain.

When we start looking for examples of ways in which pain can develop without any apparent reason, we find that there is a rare congenital disorder known as Lesch–Niehan disease in which the patient is in constant pain. This disorder is the complete opposite to the condition I have already described in which patients are not able to feel pain at all. If anything this problem is even worse; those who suffer from Lesch–Niehan disease do not survive beyond childhood but as babies struggle to scratch and tear themselves to bits.

Or consider the so-called *couvade* syndrome which has been described in many cultures around the world. In this condition it is men, not women, who suffer from labour pains or from pains of childbirth. Their wives give birth without any discomfort and return to their normal duties immediately afterwards. The husbands suffer enormous amounts of pain on behalf of their wives.

Those are extreme illustrations of the ways in which pain can exist without injury. Both are fairly rare in Western civilization. But although pain without injury may be uncommon, it is not uncommon for people to suffer from pains which are quite out of proportion to the severity of their injuries or disorders.

So, for example, take the passing of a kidney stone, a process so painful that it is often mimicked by drug addicts desperate to be given an injection of a powerful pain killer such as pethidine.

The condition begins when a kidney starts to concentrate substances normally dissolved in the urine and begins to turn those substances into tiny kidney stones. Problems usually start when a small piece breaks off one of these stones and passes into the ureter, the narrow tube that takes urine from the kidney to the bladder. As average-sized stone will be about twice as big as the normal diameter of the ureter.

Because the stone is blocking the ureter urine builds up behind it and the steadily increasing pressure means that the stone is forced further and further along the ureter towards the bladder. In order to help keep the stone moving the muscles in the wall of the ureter contract.

In purely mechanical terms the whole process is fairly trivial. The stone will only be small and the muscles involved are tiny. But the amount of pain produced by the whole incident will be entirely out of proportion. It is indeed often said that the type of pain sustained by a patient passing a kidney stone is as bad as anything a patient can ever have to endure.

In addition to those patients who sustain pains quite out of proportion to the extent of their injuries there are many patients who complain of severe pains long after their injuries have healed. Of these pains probably the most bizarre are the ones known as 'phantom limb' pains.

This phenomenon was first described by the remarkable

French father of surgery, Ambroise Paré, who in 1552 noted that after patients had had a leg cut off they would, for months afterwards, often complain of a pain not in the stump but in the leg that had been removed.

Since then phantom limb pain has been written about a great deal. In 1980, in one of the largest surveys ever done, an investigation of 29,000 American amputees found that about 2,000 were suffering from phantom limb pain. (The investigation also showed that the patients had been seen by doctors from many different medical disciplines and had, between them, received no less than forty-three different types of therapy. No one, it seems, really understands phantom limb pain.) Many of the patients were still suffering from pain in their amputated limbs long after the amputation and some time after the amputation site had completely healed. Some patients complained that they could feel pain and tingling in their missing limbs. Others complained of pains that had been present before the amputation was performed: for example, one patient who had a sliver of wood jammed under his fingernail complained of a similar pain months after his hand had been removed.

It is difficult to explain just how strange and how distressing the phenomenon of phantom limb pain can be. And it is certainly impossible to explain exactly what happens. In a way the phenomenon seems similar to what happens when, after a dental anaesthetic, we notice that our anaethetized lip feels much larger than it was before. We keep touching it and we have to go and look at ourselves in the mirror. We find it difficult to believe that the lip isn't as big as a slice of melon. But when we finally look we discover that the lip is no bigger that normal. We're imagining a sensation in an area of flesh that doesn't exist.

Common though it may be among amputees, phantom limb pain is, of course, relatively rare. There aren't all that many patients around who are unfortunate enough to have had limbs amputated.

But the phenomenon of pain existing without injury being present is neither rare nor even particularly exceptional. There are millions of people around the world who suffer from persistent and quite inexplicable pain. Approximately eight out of every ten back pain sufferers have pains which are real enough but for which no physical explanation can ever be discovered.

And of all types of pain, inexplicable pains are perhaps the most debilitating, the most tiring and the most depressing.

Hidden Influences

Next time there is an athletics meeting or a boxing match on television, take a careful look at the contestants at the end of their event or bout. The winner will look remarkably fresh and alert. He'll smile for the television cameras and answer the interviewer's questions quickly and competently. The other contestants won't look anywhere near as fit or as happy. The athletes who came in further down the field will be huffing and puffing and wheezing. The boxer who lost may well be in agony.

When the event was in progress all the athletes undoubtedly gave their best. The runners will have run as hard and as fast as they could. The boxers will have fought hard. In a 100-metre race there will be hundredths of a second separating first and second place. In a close-fought bout there may only be a narrow points decision dividing the winner from the loser. But in all cases the differences between the winner and the loser will be clearly visible. As one boxer said on television, 'It's funny with pain. It depends on whether you win or lose.'

This phenomenon isn't confined to athletes, of course. You've almost certainly experienced the same sort of thing yourself – even if you've never been near a boxing ring or an athletics track.

Perhaps you've been busy in the kitchen or the workshop and suddenly noticed that although you hadn't been aware of cutting yourself there is blood everywhere. Or maybe you've come in from an afternoon in the garden, got into the bath and suddenly found that your arms and legs are covered in scratches and bruises. Under other circumstances a small cut or a few scratches would have hurt like hell; they certainly wouldn't have gone completely unnoticed.

Those are just a few of the ways in which we feel different amounts of pain in different circumstances. It's not difficult to think of dozens of other examples. And according to the old 'specificity' theory of pain such differences were difficult, if not impossible, to explain. It's hard enough to understand why one individual should suffer less pain than another when both have identical pain receptors and nervous systems. But it sometimes seems quite impossible to understand precisely how one person can respond in so many very different ways to exactly the same series of stimuli.

Before I go on to discuss some of the hidden but specific factors which influence the way we respond to pain, and which do explain these variations, let me first add something to my original explanation of how pain produces a response.

In the earlier pages of this book I described how, when you hit yourself on the thumb, chemical changes take place which stimulate the passage of nervous impulses towards the spinal cord and eventually to the brain.

What I didn't point out on those earlier pages was that, in order for a pain to be felt, the stimulus producing the feeling must first exceed the pain threshold. In other words, if you are going to be aware that you have hit your thumb you have to have hit it with a certain amount of force. If you are very light with your hammer then you may be aware of a sensation telling you that the hammer has touched your thumb, but you won't feel a pain. You have to hit your thumb with a certain amount of force if your tissues are going to produce the chemicals necessary to stimulate a nervous response.

What is even more significant is the fact that there are not only differences between individual pain thresholds, but that pain thresholds can vary from day to day according to a wide range of hidden factors.

Nor is it just the pain threshold level that can vary; there can also be differences in the amount of pain that any individual can tolerate too. Like the pain threshold level, the pain tolerance level can be influenced by all sorts of unexpected factors. Indeed, it is our ability to tolerate, rather than simply recognize, pain that changes most of all.

On the pages which follow I have listed some of the hidden factors which have the greatest effect on your ability to tolerate pain.

Your attitude towards your pain

A patient of mine called Roger who had suffered from indigestion for some months came into my surgery and told me that his pain had suddenly got a good deal worse. I examined him carefully but could find no explanation for the change in the amount of pain he was feeling.

When I talked to Roger, however, I discovered that a friend of his had recently been diagnosed as suffering from stomach cancer. Not surprisingly, Roger was worried in case his stomach pains turned out to be caused by cancer too.

After I'd sat him down, talked to him at some length, and managed to convince him that the X-rays and other tests had all shown quite conclusively that the pains he had were not caused by stomach cancer, Roger suddenly announced that his pains had started to disappear. When I spoke to him again a few hours later he told me that the pains had gone completely.

Stories like this are common in medicine, and it seems certain that the meaning we associate with any particular pain can have an extremely important influence on the way we respond to that pain.

If we think that a pain is harmless and temporary then it will trouble us comparatively little and probably go away quite quickly. If we think that a pain signifies something threatening then the pain will stay longer and hurt more.

More than half a century ago the Russian physiologist Pavlov performed an experiment which showed just how dramatic is this link between the development of pain and the meaning we give to that pain. Having shown in previous experiments that dogs react quite violently when given strong electric shocks, Pavlov found that if he consistently gave his experimental dogs food immediately after they had been given their shocks then they would develop new responses. Immediately after an electric shock that should have been quite painful the dogs would salivate, wag their tails and turn eagerly towards their normal source of food.

Your circumstances

The point at which you start to feel pain and your ability to tolerate pain are both affected by the way in which you perceive pain and the significance that pain has for you.

One of the best examples of the way that circumstances can affect our ability to cope with pain is the way that soldiers respond to battle injuries. Way back in 1580, Montaigne wrote that 'We feel one cut from the surgeon's scalpel more than ten blows of the sword in the heat of battle.' Since then numerous observers have noticed the truth in this statement. During the Napoleonic wars, Baron Dominique-Jean Larrey, the French emperor's famous doctor, reported that soldiers seemed remarkably indifferent to battle wounds.

More recently, at the end of the Second World War, Dr Beecher, an American physician, reported that he had noticed that wounded soldiers often coped with their pain very well. Although they were severely injured they seemed to suffer very little pain. Only one out of every three seriously wounded soldiers complained of enough pain to merit being given morphine.

Moreover, Beecher reported that it wasn't that the men had become immune to any sort of pain. When given injections they still complained just as much as you or I would. But their battle wounds hardly seemed to trouble them at all.

Fascinated by his observations, Beecher asked hospital patients who had had surgery to tell him about their pain. He found that four out of every five hospital patients who had had surgery had pain bad enough to need morphine.

Leaving aside the fact that one-fifth of the hospital patients Beecher saw seemed able to cope with quite severe pain without any form of outside help, these figures are really quite remarkable. They show fairly conclusively that the circumstances in which a wound is obtained have a tremendous influence on the ability of the patient to tolerate the pain he has.

Beecher's argument to explain all this was that the wounded soldier feels some relief at being away from the battlefield. He is grateful for being alive, he has been injured in a good cause and has been fighting among friends. The ordinary hospital patient, on the other hand, will have been admitted to hospital for surgery because he is ill. He will probably be tired and frightened. He will not want to be in the hospital and he will be concerned about his future.

Incidentally, the observation that military casualties seem to feel pain far less than civilian casualties was repeated after the Yom Kippur War when a study of Israeli soldiers entirely confirmed the observations made by Montaigne, Larrey and Beecher.

Finally, more evidence to support the theory that the amount of pain an individual feels depends upon the significance of the injury causing the pain came from observations made by C. Richard Chapman, Associate Professor at the Departments of Anaesthesiology, Psychiatry and Behavioural Sciences and Psychology and the University Hospital Pain Clinic at the University of Washington, and Gary Cox, Assistant Professor at the Department of Psychiatry and Behavioural Sciences at the University of Washington.

Chapman and Cox studied patients having kidney transplants and the relatives donating the kidneys they were about to receive. They found that the amount of pain the two sets of individuals complained of varied considerably. So, for example, they found that the kidney donors complained of no pain before their surgery whereas the recipients of the kidneys did complain of pain (even though kidney disease does not necessarily cause a significant amount of pain). After surgery, however, the positions were reversed: the patients who had had surgery to remove healthy kidneys suffered considerably more pain than the patients who had received kidneys designed to save their lives. These results can easily be explained by the fact that the individuals donating kidneys had nothing to gain from the surgery – it is hardly surprising that to them the pain seemed worse.

What you're doing at the time

During a Wembley Cup Final a few years ago one of the goalkeepers broke his neck. Normally a broken neck is a pretty painful experience, and most people stop what they are doing when they break their necks. But on this occasion the goalkeeper simply took advantage of the trainer's magic sponge and carried on playing football. He was so wrapped up in the game he was playing that he didn't have time to notice the pain he was suffering. It was only when the game was finished that he suddenly realized that he was in agony.

That story may sound rather extreme but it does illustrate a very common experience. If you're busy with an important golf match you probably won't notice that you've acquired blisters on three fingers. If you're involved in a tennis match that you're really enjoying then you won't notice that you've sprained your shoulder or grazed your knee badly. Our ability to tolerate pain goes up dramatically when we're busy doing something that has attracted our attention.

The 'something' doesn't have to be anything sporting, of course. It can be anything that attracts and holds your attention for long enough.

In an experiment conducted in 1963, three researchers found that they were able to increase the pain tolerance levels of a group of volunteers if they allowed their volunteers to listen to music, tap their feet and sing out loud. When subjected to pain with no chance to distract themselves the pain tolerance levels of the volunteers were quite low. When allowed to 'lose' themselves in music the volunteers managed to tolerate much greater amounts of pain.

Incidentally, research has also shown that distraction works best if the pain is kept steady or if it rises fairly slowly. A pain that suddenly appears or changes in intensity quite quickly will be much more difficult to ignore.

Whether you're an introvert or an extrovert

During the 1970s quite a number of researchers investigated the theory that shy, quiet individuals are likely to have lower pain tolerance levels than abrasive, noisy, extroverted characters.

In 1976, for example, Curt Bartol and Nancy Costello of Castleton State College in the United States of America concluded that 'extroverted personalities . . . are more tolerant of pain than introverted personalities', while in 1975, Gordon Barnes of York University, Ontario in Canada concluded that the results produced by several research teams around the world 'strongly support the contention that introverts are less tolerant of pain' and that 'extroverts have higher pain thresholds and show greater pain tolerance than introverts'.

The available evidence does, therefore, seem to substantiate the theory that extroverts have higher pain thresholds and greater pain tolerance than introverts.

How frightened you are

Have you ever had toothache, booked an appointment to see the dentist, and found that by the time you walked into his consulting room your pain had disappeared?

You aren't alone if you've experienced something like this. It's an extremely common happening. And it has nothing to do with the body's innate ability to heal itself.

The simple explanation is that when we start to be aware of an aching tooth our threshold is fairly low. We are worried by the pain and we don't know how long it is going to last. Nor do we know when we are likely to be able to get an appointment to see a dentist for advice and treatment. Our natural fears ensure that our pain threshold and tolerance remain low.

As soon as we've booked the appointment with the dentist, however, our anxiety begins to lift. We feel more confident about having the problem dealt with. We realize that we only have to put up with the problem for a finite length of time. Because we know that relief will soon be at hand we suffer far less from the pain.

Toothache isn't the only type of pain to be adversely

affected by uncertainty, fear and anxiety, of course. Any type of fear or anxiety will make any pain much worse.

One of the most interesting pieces of research to link anxiety and pain was done in 1954 when two researchers found that if they gave volunteers small electric shocks without mentioning the word 'pain' beforehand, the volunteers did not regard the shocks as painful. If, however, the word 'pain' was mentioned before the shocks were given, many of the volunteers complained that the shocks were painful.

Whether you're depressed

If you've ever had a day when you've felt really depressed then you'll know just how a depression can affect your whole life and your way of dealing with problems.

If you're feeling on top of the world and a shirt button comes off or a shoelace breaks, you'll probably think nothing of it. You'll reach for the needle and thread or a clean shirt, and you'll either make do with half a shoelace or you'll find a spare one. The problem won't make much of a dent in your day.

If, however, you're feeling really miserable when a shirt button comes off then you'll probably burst into tears. Your response will be out of all proportion.

The way we respond to pain is influenced by our mood in exactly the same sort of way. If you're feeling unhappy and you hit your thumb then the pain may stay with you all day long. Indeed, the pain may well exacerbate your depression, with the inevitable result that you become locked in a vicious circle. Your pain will make your depression worse; your depression will make you more susceptible to pain, and as your pain threshold is lowered so your depression will be deepened.

What you learned as a child

Children are, it seems, deeply influenced by the attitudes of their parents towards pain. If a child's parents make a tremendous fuss over him every time he gets a knock or bruise then when that child grows up he will have a comparatively low pain threshold and low tolerance level. If, however, a child's parents take little notice when he complains then he will grow up fairly indifferent to pain, with a higher pain threshold and a greater ability to tolerate pain.

There is also evidence to suggest that children may 'learn' specific types of pain behaviour from their parents too. So, for example, half the children who get recurrent abdominal pain for which no explanation can be found come from families where a close relative has a similar type of pain, while young girls whose mothers regularly complain of period pains are far more likely to grow up suffering period pains themselves than are girls whose mothers do not complain of period pains.

How happy you were when you were small

In 1978 the journal *Pain* published a report from Drs H. Merskey and D. Boyd of the Department of Psychiatry at the University of Western Ontario and the London Psychiatric Hospital, also in Ontario, which showed that children who have unhappy childhoods are likely to grow up more vulnerable to pain than children who have happy, well-balanced childhoods.

After examining 141 patients suffering from chronic pain Merskey and Boyd also concluded that patients whose marriages have been unhappy are more at risk too.

Your race and nationality

The nationality of an individual has a tremendous effect on his or her ability to tolerate pain. The Italians and the Indians seem to have a low pain tolerance level, while the English (particularly English males) value a 'stiff upper lip' and have a high pain tolerance level. Jews seem less capable of coping with pain than Gentiles, while in general Northern Europeans and Americans of Northern European extraction tend to be rather stoical and capable of tolerating greater amounts of pain.

The variations in racial susceptibility to pain were perhaps best shown by a survey of over 40,000 patients that was carried out by Drs Kenneth Woodrow, Gary Friedman, A. B. Siegelaub and Morris Collen. Each patient was given a simple pain tolerance test in which the amount of pressure he could tolerate was measured, with the pressure being gradually increased until the patient told the researcher to stop.

The results showed that the whites had the highest average pain tolerance. Blacks came second. Surprisingly, perhaps, it turned out that the traditional picture of a stoical Oriental is something of a myth. The Japanese and Chinese came third in this study.

The size of your family

The size of the family in which a child grows up can have a tremendous influence on the child's eventual pain threshold and pain tolerance levels.

One of the earliest pieces of research to substantiate this observation was published in 1970 by Donald Sweeney and Bernard Fine of the United States Army Research Institute of Environmental Medicine. The two researchers tested the abilities of a group of volunteers to withstand pain, and found that children who grow up with at least three other brothers and sisters are likely to have much higher pain tolerance levels than children who grow up with fewer brothers and sisters.

Since then other researchers have shown that 'only' children are likely to grow up with lower pain threshold and tolerance levels than anyone. This is, in fact, hardly surprising since 'only' children are far more likely to receive constant, high levels of sympathy and attention from their parents.

Your age

Our ability to tolerate pain changes as we get older; we become better able to tolerate superficial skin pains and less able to tolerate deeper pains.

Your sex

In a number of research projects conducted around the world it has been found that although women have much the same sort of pain threshold as men, they are less tolerant of pain than are men. S. L. H. Notermans and M. M. W. A. Tophoff of the State University in Gronigen, The Netherlands published a paper as long ago as 1967 in which they concluded that men can tolerate pain better than women. They could find no physiological explanation for this discovery, but argued that men are taught to be 'stronger' than women and that it is less socially acceptable for a man to cry out in pain than it is for a woman to cry out in pain.

In another, more recent experiment conducted by Thomas Wescott, Lorrie Huesz, Donald Boswell and Patricia Herold, all of Pennsylvania State University, it was shown that men can tolerate pain for 20 per cent longer than women.

In possibly the largest experiment of its kind ever conducted, four American physicians from California concluded that although pain tolerance often falls with age, older men have a higher pain tolerance than younger women.

Your attitude towards health

If you worry about your health a great deal, you are likely to have a fairly low tolerance for pain.

Dr David Nichols and Bernard Turksy from the Department of Psychiatry at Harvard Medical School in Boston examined thirty male college students psychologically and then tested them for pain sensitivity. They found that the students who were most anxious about their bodies were least able to tolerate pain.

And finally . . .

Disabled teenage girl Terrie Hayes, who has had both legs amputated below the knee, was one of twenty-four brave youngsters who attended the 1985 Barnardo's Champion Children of the Year Award Ceremony at the Savoy Hotel in London.

Terrie, who met Princess Diana at the ceremony, said afterwards, 'I can't remember a thing we talked about. But talking to the Princess made me forget the pain.'

PART TWO

Doctors, Drugs, Surgery and Alternative Medicine

Doctors and Pain

Pain is the biggest single problem doctors have to face. It causes more misery, more unhappiness and more depression than all other symptoms put together. It ruins the lives of millions and wrecks careers, friendships and marriages.

When left unrelieved pain leads to physical and mental exhaustion, to disablement and to chronic anxiety. Patients with pain are likely to develop medical complications, likely to need additional medical treatment and likely to need to spend lengthy periods in hospital. People get better slower when they are in pain, and they need more support both from friends and relatives and from the professionals.

And yet, sadly, the majority of doctors are not very good at dealing with pain. Speaking at the Third World Congress on Pain, Dr Robert Twycross, a consultant at the Churchill Hospital in Oxford, and one of the world's leading experts on pain relief, claimed that up to three-quarters of patients with persistent pain get poor treatment from their doctors.

Other eminent experts have made equally damning observations. And millions of patients would confirm that although their doctors may seem to do all that they can, their abilities to control pain are, to put it mildly, unsatisfactory. As one cynic put it, 'Doctors are very good at tolerating other people's pain.'

At first sight it may seem difficult to understand why this should be. Doctors have, after all, dedicated their lives to the relief of suffering. But in fact there are several very good reasons why doctors are so bad at treating pain.

First, and perhaps most important, medical schools spend very little time teaching students about pain or about pain relief. The majority of practising doctors will have never heard of the gate control theory of pain; they will have been taught a little about pain receptors and nervous pathways but virtually nothing about techniques for relieving pain. Academic doctors (the type who teach in medical schools) like to think of medicine as a scientific discipline, and they prefer to encourage students to search for permanent cures rather than to spend time offering symptomatic relief. If they were to emphasize the treatment of pain the professors would have to admit that medicine does not have all the answers and cannot always produce specific diagnoses or offer specific cures. Astonishingly, a 1983 survey of seventeen standard textbooks on medicine, surgery and cancer found that out of 22,000 pages only fifty-four provided any information at all about pain. Half the standard medical textbooks didn't discuss pain at all. Even quasi-academic organizations which ought to be concerned with pain seem to prefer to put their energies into searching only for cures; in America, for example, the National Cancer Institute spends little more than 0.2 per cent of its annual budget on pain research. Most frightening of all is the fact that for most doctors education stops when they leave medical school, and what postgraduate education they receive is dominated by the drug industry.

Second, because doctors are taught so little about ways of relieving pain, they become extremely frustrated when faced with a seemingly endless queue of patients who have persistent, troublesome pains for which no cause can be found. The medical academics who are buried in their medical schools may be able to hide from reality, but the doctor in practice has to deal with hundreds of patients who are in pain and who need help. For the practising physician there is no escape.

Doctors respond to their own feelings of frustration and inadequacy in a number of ways. Some spend their working lives searching for solutions, trying out new theories and offering their own favourite remedies. Sadly, because they know so little about the ways in which pain is produced, many of the doctors searching for cures offer remedies which are of very little real value.

Others, often tetchy and irritable and consumed by

professional guilt, merely pass such patients on to colleagues, putting patients onto the world's most expensive merry-go-round. 'This isn't my speciality,' says the psychiatrist, 'you need to see a surgeon.' 'This isn't my sort of problem,' says the surgeon, 'you need to see a psychiatrist.' Dr C. Norman Shealy, the eminent and sensible American neurosurgeon has reported seeing one patient who had had no less than forty operations on his back. The cost for all the operations came to just under half a million dollars.

Third, because they have learnt so little about the ways in which pain can be produced and made worse, doctors often tend to offer quite inappropriate advice. For example, many doctors encourage patients who complain of pain to 'take things easy' and to 'stay in bed'. All the available evidence suggests that such traditional advice is likely to make things worse rather than better. Doctors will also often turn to drugs as a first line of attack for pain, not necessarily because drugs are best, but simply because they will have received all their postgraduate training from drug companies anxious to sell their products. For ten years now a few independent researchers (many of them psychologists rather than doctors) have been searching for, identifying and testing new ways of dealing with pain. Many of the techniques they have discovered are effective, safe and inexpensive. But the drug companies have no interest in such non-drug therapies and so practising doctors, who don't have the time, the training or the inclination to read through the world's medical literature, accept what they are told by drug company representatives.

All this means that most pain sufferers might as well be living in underdeveloped countries. And until those who run our medical schools and postgraduate training courses realize how important pain relief is, and how many people need help and advice, then the majority of pain sufferers will receive inadequate support from their doctors.

That is the sad and depressing news about pain management. The good news is that in the last ten years researchers have discovered a number of ways of dealing with pain and of providing help for those sufferers in need. All the techniques they have investigated and described can be used, quite safely, without professional medical help. Freedom from pain may still be a dream. But it is now possible for every individual to learn how to control his or her pain. And the Pain Control Programme which takes up the greater part of this book is designed to help you do just that.

But before we reach the Pain Control Programme I would like to discuss those medical and surgical techniques which *are* available, in some greater depth. For, although the medical profession has relatively little to offer many pain sufferers, there are times when a doctor's advice must be sought. And if you know what doctors can – and cannot – do, then you will be in a much better position to take advantage of medical skills.

Drugs

For most people drugs are still the commonest way of dealing with pain. The majority of doctors will write out a prescription for pain killers whenever they see patients complaining of pain. And there are scores of different products available for them to choose from.

Similarly, there are scores of pain-killing products available to patients to buy for themselves. When I wrote my book *The Medicine Men* just a few years ago drug companies were producing 2,000 tons of aspirin every year for consumption in Britain alone – and selling those aspirin tablets under no less than 104 different trade names. Today the market is even bigger. In an average sort of year the British buy about three billion pain-killing tablets and pay out around £80 million for them. The annual sales of pain killers in chemists' shops and supermarkets rise every year.

Traditionally, many different products have been used for providing pain relief. At various times in history such plants as hemp, hemlock, henbane and mandrake have all been popular. Today, however, the two types of drug considered most effective and used most widely are the products which were traditionally extracted from the willow tree and the poppy: aspirin and morphine. Today 99 per cent of all the drugs used as pain killers come from one or other of these two drug families.

The aspirin family

The effectiveness of acetylsalicylic acid (the drug first extracted from the willow) was first described in a scientific paper some 200 years ago, but it wasn't until the end of the nineteenth century that tablets called 'aspirin' came on to the market and were made readily available in chemists' shops.

The salicylates may be the most popular drugs to have come from the willow tree but during the last few decades chemists have taken many more products from the same basic source. Drugs such as phenylbutazone, paracetamol, phenacetin, indomethacin, mefanamic acid and ibuprofen all come from the same original plant as the common or garden aspirin tablet.

Although we still don't really know how any of these drugs work we do know that they suppress inflammation, pain and fever with varying degrees of effectiveness and with varying side effects. The most likely explanation is that drugs such as aspirin block the synthesis of prostaglandins, the chemicals which are produced when bodily tissues are damaged and which have the job of producing localized swelling and stimulating the nerve endings to send pain messages to the brain.

Naturally aspirin and all the other drugs in this group can cause a number of side effects, sometimes even when prescribed in fairly modest quantities. The commonest problem associated with aspirin is gastric irritation and bleeding, but among other side effects patients may also complain of dizziness and ringing in their ears if they take too many aspirin tablets. There are some patients who are sensitive to all the products in this group and can't take any of them without feeling uncomfortable or developing unpleasant allergy symptoms.

The existence of these side effects has, however, been overemphasized in the last few years. Aspirin tablets can prove lethal, but the dangers have been exaggerated by drug companies anxious to sell alternative products. The problem with simple, old-fashioned aspirin is that the patent doesn't belong to any single drug company and, since there are so many companies making the product, the price is very low. It's difficult to get rich out of selling your own variation on this traditional theme.

Because of this, numerous companies have in recent years introduced their own alternative pain killers. For sale 'over the counter' companies have produced and then promoted products containing both aspirin and paracetamol, and products containing aspirin and the stimulant caffeine. Many companies have simply wrapped up quite ordinary aspirin tablets in expensive packaging and sold them with the aid of convincing advertising programmes. The one useful advance that has been made has involved the development of soluble aspirin tablets which can be swallowed in liquid form rather than as tablets. Research evidence has shown quite conclusively that soluble aspirin tablets are far less likely to cause stomach irritation and are therefore safer than the ordinary, old-fashioned non-soluble type.

Because doctors are slightly more difficult to dupe than ordinary customers, the drug companies have been rather more sophisticated in their attempts to introduce new prescription-only pain killers designed to take the place of the traditional aspirin tablet. They have used all sorts of clever tricks to help them convince doctors of the value of their latest product. One trick, for example, has been to produce a new 'alternative' drug and then to measure its effectiveness and likelihood of producing side effects against that of ordinary insoluble aspirin. Since the insoluble aspirin tablet is particularly likely to produce gastric irritation it isn't difficult to show that the new product is less dangerous. If the company had compared its product with soluble aspirin then the results would have probably been far less flattering.

During the last few decades an extraordinary number of alternative pain killers have been launched, promoted and prescribed. Many have been specifically designed for use with patients suffering from diseases such as arthritis and backache – both problems which affect millions of patients and which tend to persist for many years.

Unhappily, however, a remarkable number of these aspirin 'alternatives' have lasted only a year or two before having to be removed from the market as too dangerous. Time and time again a product has been put on to the market, prescribed in huge quantities and then removed when it has become clear that the drug is neither as effective as aspirin nor as safe.

Other drugs have been put on to the market and have maintained their popularity despite a lack of any genuine evidence to prove their superiority over aspirin. So, for example, despite the safety, effectiveness and cheapness of aspirin, for years one of the drugs most commonly prescribed for the treatment of pain was a proprietary product called Distalgesic. Doctors prescribed it in huge quantities because they believed that it was stronger and yet safer than aspirin. If the doctors who prescribed Distalgesic so enthusiastically had done their homework they would have found no conclusive evidence to show that the drug was any better than aspirin, but they would have found evidence that it is chemically similar to the synthetic opiate methadone. Only after Distalgesic had been prescribed by thousands of doctors for millions of patients was it finally realized that the drug was addictive.

The opiates

The other important group of pain-killing drugs are the opiates – drugs originally extracted from the opium poppy and including such well-known pain killers as morphine and heroin.

The history of these drugs goes back a long, long way. Opium was known to the Sumerians nearly six thousand years ago. Hippocrates, the father of modern medicine, prescribed opium too, and the great Roman physician Galen used it for relieving pain.

By the nineteenth century opium had become probably the most popular drug in the world and it was widely used throughout Europe. The British fought the Chinese for the right to continue exporting opium to China, and in the single year 1870 a staggering 90,000 pounds of opium were officially and quite legally imported into Britain.

There are, of course, almost as many variations on the opium theme as there are on the aspirin theme. Opium itself contains about 10 per cent morphine and rather smaller amounts of other substances, including one called codeine which is related to morphine. From these basic constituents a number of products have been prepared which vary in potency, duration of effect and the number of side effects they produce. All are similar in that they produce a fairly considerable amount of pain relief and tend to make patients feel sleepy.

Although it has been recognized for thousands of years that the opiates are extremely effective as pain killers it has only been in the last decade that scientists have managed to work out exactly how the opiates work. And the explanation is both fascinating and revealing: morphine and heroin work simply and solely because they imitate twenty or so natural hormones, the endorphins and enkephalins, which are produced within the brain and which are the body's own special answers to pain.

It was in Scotland in the 1970s that some of the earliest work was done. Two research pharmacologists at the University of Aberdeen, John Hughes and Hans Kosterlitz, succeeded in isolating previously unknown, powerful pain-blocking chemicals that occur naturally in the brain and the spinal cord. Hughes and Kosterlitz found that these naturally occurring hormones, now known as endorphins, can switch off the body's pain alarm by fitting into special receptors on nerve cells.

The body produces these internal pain-killing hormones when it needs to overcome pain in order to survive. So, for example, if a soldier has injured his ankle but is being chased by enemy soldiers then his body will numb the pain of his damaged ankle with its internally-produced endorphins so that he will be able to keep running and save his own life. Those same endorphins are also produced when we are busy doing something that our minds consider more important than 'pain'. If you're playing tennis in an important match and you injure your arm then your body will produce endorphins so that you can ignore the pain. Only when the match is over will the endorphin production cease and will you become aware of the pain.

Morphine and heroin, the drugs we think of as the most powerful pain killers available are, in fact, merely counterfeit endorphins. They achieve their effect by interacting with those natural receptors and by imitating the effect of the body's own natural pain-killing hormones.

Because, in addition to their pain-killing qualities, the

opiates also have an effect on the mood of the person taking them, these drugs have in recent years been involved in a good deal of controversy. A number of people have become addicted to morphine and heroin and both these two drugs – but particularly heroin – have become popular with pushers of illegal drugs. The addiction problems associated with these drugs have led to two specific problems associated with the role of opiates as pain relievers.

First, there has been controversy over whether or not doctors should be allowed to prescribe heroin for pain relief. About thirty years ago the World Health Organization suggested that in order to help control the drug addiction problem heroin should be banned completely. Doctors in just about every country in the world accepted this suggestion (heroin was banned in the United States in 1956) – but doctors in Britain refused to cooperate and insisted on retaining the right to prescribe heroin. Many experts now believe that it was Britain's refusal to cooperate which helped contribute to the current epidemic of heroin abuse. The problem is now being made much worse by the fact that because doctors in Britain have continued to use heroin doctors in other countries (and in particular America) are now demanding the right to prescribe the drug too.

In fact, the evidence now available largely suggests that British doctors were quite wrong to fight for the right to continue prescribing heroin. One of the world's leading experts in the treatment of pain is Dr Robert Twycross, who has worked at St Christopher's Hospice in London and the Churchill Hospital, Oxford. In several articles Dr Twycross has managed to show that neither patients nor doctors can observe any difference between morphine and heroin. This conclusion is supported by research work done by Stanley Wallenstein and his associates at the Memorial Sloan Kettering Cancer Center in New York. Dr Wallenstein's study involved 124 cancer patients with post-operative pain and another forty-six with chronic pain, and showed that heroin is neither better nor worse than morphine.

The second problem associated with the use of morphine and heroin in pain relief is much more serious, but is a direct consequence of the fact that these drugs have become popular drugs of addiction. Because they are worried about their patients becoming addicted to these pain-relieving drugs, many doctors are reluctant to prescribe these chemicals in large enough quantities, and equally reluctant to allow their patients to take the drugs for the length of time they need them. The inevitable result is that many patients suffering from severe and persistent pain have been left in agony.

In fact, the available evidence shows quite conclusively that it is extremely rare for patients who use opiates to relieve pain to become addicted. In a survey made of thousands of Israeli casualties in the Yom Kippur War it was found that although many of the wounded soldiers had been given morphine not one of them had become addicted. Similar evidence was produced by American doctors working with soldiers fighting in Vietnam and has been duplicated by other physicians working with patients suffering from pain. It seems clear that patients suffering from pain can stop taking opiates without any adverse effects if their pain disappears or can be controlled in some other way. These conclusions fit in well with the philosophy that claims that it is the personality of the individual and his circumstances and expectations which determine whether or not he becomes an addict, and not simply the nature of the drug he is taking. However, with drugs such as the benzodiazepines (see below) this relationship is clouded by the fact that the drugs produce symptoms such as anxiety and depression and thereby adversely affect both the individual's personality and his expectations.

Tranquillizers

The aspirin type of drugs and the opiates are the two most popularly prescribed pain-killing products. But there is a third type of drug widely used by doctors when dealing with patients suffering from persistent or recurrent pain: the tranquillizers, and in particular the group of drugs known as the benzodiazepines.

First introduced in the early 1960s, the benzodiazepines include a number of well-known branded products. In the few years since then these drugs have become the most widely-used prescription drugs in the world, and by wildly overprescribing them doctors have produced the world's biggest drug addiction problem.

These products were originally designed to be used as short-term aids for patients suffering from anxiety, but many doctors use them as multi-purpose drugs and hand them out to patients for whom they can think of no more specific product. There are two definite reasons why doctors have commonly prescribed the benzodiazepines for patients suffering from pain. First, patients who suffer regularly from pain are often anxious and depressed and they frequently have difficulty in getting to sleep at night. And second, doctors simply do not know how else to treat such patients. In their frustration they turn to the benzodiazepines which tend to make patients sleepy, more cooperative and less complaining.

The major problem with the benzodiazepines is, of course, not just that they produce all sorts of unpleasant and potentially dangerous side effects but that after a few weeks they make people feel anxious and depressed (these are the very symptoms for which they are commonly prescribed, even though they are not recommended for the treatment of depression), and are extremely addictive. They are, indeed, believed to be among the most addictive drugs of all. Testifying to a United States Senate health subcommittee in Washington in 1979, one expert said even then that tranquillizers provided America's number one drug problem apart from alcohol. Another expert reported that it is harder to 'kick' the tranquillizer habit than it is to get off heroin.

Despite these important hazards the majority of doctors continue to prescribe benzodiazepines in huge quantities. In Britain in 1986 there were estimated to be 2½ million benzodiazepine addicts – many of them pain sufferers.

According to the scientific evidence which is now available patients would be better off if they were given heroin. For not only are the benzodiazepines dangerously addictive, but they are also worse than useless for patients suffering from pain. In an experiment conducted by four researchers in Missouri, led by John Stern of the Behavior Research Laboratory at Washington University, diazepam (the most widely prescribed of all benzodiazepines) was shown to make some patients more sensitive to pain.

Getting the best out of drugs

There is no doubt that drugs can make extremely effective weapons in the battle against pain. But sadly, drugs are not always used wisely or effectively. In a survey of 800 patients who attended the Oxford Regional Pain Unit 14 per cent had given up taking drugs that had been prescribed for them because they felt that they weren't deriving any benefit from them. An even larger group were still taking their drugs but were prepared to admit that they were deriving no benefit from drugs at all. These figures strongly suggest not only that drugs should be considered only as part of a wider programme to control pain, but also that many doctors who treat patients suffering from pain do not properly understand how drugs should be used. I feel that the answer is for patients themselves to take a greater interest in the drugs they are given and to learn enough to be able to offer constructive, practical advice to their own physicians.

The first thing to remember is that there are really only three useful drugs for the treatment of pain: aspirin, codeine and morphine. There are literally hundreds of alternative pain-killing drugs available, but there is no evidence to show that any of the alternatives are better than these three simple products. Those patients who cannot take aspirin because they are sensitive to it can substitute paracetamol, but otherwise there is little point in trying any variations on these themes. Indeed, there are many experts who would claim that there are really only two drugs worth using: aspirin and morphine; and that any pain that cannot be controlled by an acceptable dose of aspirin needs treatment with morphine.

If a pain cannot be relieved by ordinary soluble aspirin then it is much more sensible to try increasing the dose of aspirin than to try switching to an alternative but basically similar product. If, when the maximum dose of aspirin has been reached, the pain has still not been controlled, then the only pharmacological solution is to change to morphine.

Second, if you are going to take a drug, it is important to take the drug in a large enough quantity. It has been well known for some years that one of the main reasons why so many patients fail to get proper relief from the drugs they are taking is that they are not taking their drugs in large enough doses. In a now famous study carried out in 1973 two psychiatrists, Richard Marks and Edward Sachar of New York City's Montefiore Hospital, found that nearly three-quarters of hospital patients receiving opiates for moderate to severe pain failed to get relief from the drugs they were taking.

Surprised by this, Marks and Sachar investigated further and discovered that the patients had been prescribed only one-half to three-quarters of the required dosage. Furthermore, they discovered that the nurses who gave the drugs and the injections had in practice reduced the drug levels even more. As a result some patients were getting less than one-quarter of the medication they really needed.

Leaving aside the possibility that all the doctors and nurses concerned were sadists, the only conclusion that could be drawn from this study was that the doctors in charge of these patients had underestimated the extent of their patients' pain, overestimated the power of the drugs they were prescribing, and worried too much about the danger of their patients becoming addicted.

If you're going to take a drug there is no point in taking it unless you get proper pain relief. If the drug doesn't help you then keep asking your doctor to increase the dosage.

Third, anyone taking a drug should not wait until his pain has returned before taking his next dose. That is not a sign of strength, it is a sign of ignorance. By only taking a drug when you are in terrible pain you will be weakening your body, and by learning to associate your drug with pain relief you will be making yourself more dependent on drug relief than you would be if you took your pills at regular times. According to Dr Mark Swerdlow and Dr Jan Stjernswärd, both of the World Health Organization Cancer Unit, pain-killing drugs should be given according to the clock and not according to the presence or absence of pain. They claim that each successive dose should be taken before the effects of the previous dose have worn off and before the pain has returned, and argue that, if this philosophy is followed, the amount of pain killer required can be kept to a minimum and gradually reduced. Other experts agree with them.

Surgery

When the traditional Descartes theory of pain transmission was still popular (see page 13) surgeons decided that they ought to be able to help patients suffering from persistent or recurrent pain either by destroying the nerves carrying messages from the body to the brain, or by destroying those parts of the brain suspected to be responsible for receiving and interpreting messages about pain.

As a result they created a number of apparently sophisticated surgical operations designed to help patients suffering from pain. They devised ways of destroying nerves by injecting them with toxic substances; they worked out ways in which they could burn nerves with electricity or destroy them by freezing. And they thought up all sorts of brain operations which they believed would help prevent patients from feeling pain. Neurosurgery became one of the fastest growing of all surgical specialities, and at one time it was said that if a patient in America complained of a headache he'd probably find himself being operated on by a neurosurgeon before he even had time to reach for a bottle of aspirin tablets.

Melzack and Wall, the two researchers who devised the gate control theory, once told a terrifying story about a man who developed a pain in one of his arms. To start with surgeons amputated the man's arm. When that failed they performed two more operations to cut the nerves which had supplied the arm. They then followed up with two operations on the frontal lobes of the man's brain. Unhappily, although these operations affected the man's mind, they still didn't get rid of the pain and so another operation was performed to destroy yet another part of his brain. The pain still hadn't disappeared and the much-mutilated patient then committed suicide.

During the 1960s and 1970s thousands of patients suffering from persistent or recurrent pain were operated on by neurosurgeons. And thousands of patients were badly and permanently mutilated. My own view is that neurosurgeons are probably the cruellest, least useful and most destructive of all surgeons. There are still many thousands of them around the world, often earning huge fees from operating on patients whose lives are so destroyed with pain that they will accept any hope, however slender. The real tragedy is, of course, that pain is affected by an enormous range of different factors. It involves emotion, experiences, expectations and fears. Physiology and psychology are intertwined in a way we still don't properly understand. Trying to deal with persistent pain by cutting nerves or chopping out chunks of brain is about as subtle and reliable as kicking a television set that isn't working properly, and about as logical as tearing the innards out of your motor car when it won't start. There are good and sensible neurosurgeons around but they are far outnumbered by the crude, the thoughtless and the ignorant. Countless patients who have been operated on by neurosurgeons are now in far more pain and far more distress than they ever were before.

Even the one fairly minor procedure that was popular among neurosurgeons in the late 1960s and early 1970s, and which involved implanting an electrode into the spinal cord so that the patient could use an external transmitter to stimulate his nerves directly whenever he was suffering from pain, has now been discredited. Dorsal column stimulation (or DCS as it was known for short) was originally hailed as a revolutionary, safe and effective way of relieving otherwise intractable pain without permanently destroying nerves.

But when, in the early 1980s, Drs D. L. Erickson and D. M. Long reassessed eighty patients who had undergone the operation at the University of Minnesota Hospitals between 1970 and 1975 they came to the conclusion that a good deal of the success attributed to dorsal column stimulation owed more to the enthusiasm of the surgeon than to the benefits enjoyed by the patient. According to Dr Erickson's figures the long-term success rate of the operation was no higher than 3 per cent.

Today, many responsible neurosurgeons seem to spend more time persuading their patients not to have surgery than they do operating. When a surgeon cuts nerves or removes pieces of brain, he is damaging delicate tissues irreversibly and the risks are enormous.

Any patient whose pain is so severe and so untreatable that he is prepared to consider surgery should ask himself a series of quite simple questions:

1. What is the worst that can happen to me if I do not have this operation? Can my condition get worse? How likely is it that my condition will get worse?

2. What do I stand to gain from this operation? What is the very best that the surgeon can offer me? And what are the chances of the operation being that successful?

3. What are the risks of the operation? What can go wrong? And what are the chances of something going wrong?

4. What alternative solutions are there that I still have not tried? What are the risks with these alternative solutions?

Pain Clinics

During World War II Dr John Bonica was chief of anaesthesiology at a military hospital where the 7,700 beds were regularly filled with soldiers suffering from serious war wounds and injuries. Each day the young anaesthetist found himself struggling to find ways to help relieve the awful pain of the men in his care. Desperate for information, he started consulting other specialists at the hospital and talking to anyone who could offer him information about the best ways of dealing with pain.

It was that wartime experience which led Dr Bonica to develop the concept of the pain clinic. His hope was that doctors would be able to work together, learn about pain and its treatment, try out new techniques and gradually accumulate experience and information which could be used to help other patients. The idea was an excellent one, but sadly most of the pain clinics in existence today consist of nothing but a single doctor who has been lumbered with the job of looking after the patients no other specialist can be bothered with. The pain clinic in many modern hospitals is the dumping ground for patients whose problems cannot be sorted out and for whom no cure seems possible.

In too many hospitals the term 'pain clinic' has been used to add dignity and hope to an outpatients department with a long waiting list where a single overworked specialist offers patients a straight choice between drug therapy and surgery.

In 1982 Dr J. W. Lloyd of the Pain Relief Unit at Abingdon Hospital in Oxfordshire reported in the *Journal of the Royal Society of Medicine* that in the United Kingdom no less than 95 per cent of all pain clinics are run by anaesthetists, often working single-handed. In 1984 the Director of the Centre for Pain Relief at Walton Hospital in Liverpool reported that 'At our clinic, possibly the largest in the country, there is now an eighteen-month waiting list for patients with chronic back pain. . . .'

It has been said that although pain is everyone's business it is no one's responsibility, and it seems to me that the existence of pain clinics is used by many doctors as yet another excuse for avoiding responsibility.

Alternative Medicine

Discouraged by the failure of the medical profession to offer any real solutions to their problems, many patients suffering from persistent or recurrent pain have turned to alternative practitioners. There are today thousands of practitioners working in dozens of different specialities who are offering advice and help to patients suffering from pain. I have here chosen to illustrate the points I want to make by referring only to two of the commonest: acupuncture and hypnotherapy.

Acupuncture

Acupuncture has been used in China for around 4,000 years. It was first made popular in Europe by a Dutch physician called Willem ten Rhyne who introduced it into Holland in 1683, but since then it has been 'rediscovered' by Western doctors every few decades or so. In some countries, such as France, there are now acupuncture departments in many major hospitals. In other countries, such as Britain, acupuncture is still regarded by many doctors as a quack remedy that shouldn't really be taken seriously. In some countries you have to be a qualified doctor before you're allowed to practise acupuncture. In other countries you can practise acupuncture without any officially-recognized qualifications whatsoever. In Britain, for example, you can put up a brass plate and describe yourself as an acupuncturist with absolutely no training at all.

The theory upon which the practice of acupuncture is founded is that the human body contains twelve main meridians or channels along which vital internal energies flow. When these meridians are blocked in some way the flow of energy is impeded and the individual becomes ill or develops a pain.

The practice of acupuncture is built upon the suggestion that there are a number of specific points on the human body which can be regarded as entrances or exits for this internal energy force. As long ago as the fourteenth century Chinese doctors had identified no fewer than 657 acupuncture points. Today over 1,000 acupuncture points have been identified.

In order to use these acupuncture points to clear blocked meridians and relieve pain, the acupuncturist uses slender needles made of pure silver, gold or copper. After first making a diagnosis about the cause of the pain (obtained in traditional acupuncture style by talking and listening to the patient and by checking the twelve different pulses which Chinese doctors claim they can identify), the acupuncturist inserts his needles and then manipulates them by one of several quite separate, principal techniques.

In the first the acupuncturist inserts his needle and twists it backwards and forwards vigorously for a few seconds. This is usually a rather painful experience. In the second he inserts his needle or needles and leaves it (or them) in place for some twenty or thirty minutes. Occasionally he may connect the needles to an apparatus which passes a mild electric current through them. Sometimes he may dry and shred leaves of the Chinese wormwood plant and then burn these shredded leaves directly over an acupuncture point (this is known as moxibustion). As a final alternative the acupuncturist may search out tender trigger points and then insert his needles into those specific areas.

There is no doubt that acupuncture works and is particularly effective for the treatment of pain. Back in 1974 four American surgeons reported that they had treated over 300 patients in and around the New York area by acupuncture. The surgeons stated that in over three-quarters of the cases they had found that acupuncture is one of the most effective treatments available for skeletomuscular disorders such as arthritis. Two doctors writing in the *Canadian Anesthetists' Society Journal* in the same year wrote that 'Reports of a large number of surgical cases operated on under acupuncture anaesthesia with a success rate of up to 90 per cent have now been sufficiently substantiated that the effectiveness of acupuncture can no longer be doubted.' By 1979 acupuncture had been so widely tested that at a meeting of medical representatives from all six of the World Health Organization's regions it was concluded that 'The sheer weight of evidence demands that it must be taken seriously as a clinical procedure of considerable value.' All sorts of silly claims have been made for acupuncture, but the evidence now available suggests that it is a powerful and effective way of dealing with pain in something like 70 per cent of all cases.

The main reason why acupuncture has never really caught on among doctors is, of course, the fact that it has always been difficult to explain exactly how acupuncture works. Doctors are notoriously cautious about accepting new methods of treatment that they don't understand.

Today there is at last evidence which shows precisely how acupuncture works, and the real irony is that this new evidence now makes it almost certain that acupuncture will never become an accepted form of medical treatment. By learning how acupuncture works we have learned how to obtain the same sort of effect without using the needles.

It seems that at least two things happen when a needle is pushed into the skin. First, by introducing a sensation into the skin which passes along the larger nerve fibres and closes the gate in the spinal cord, acupuncture prevents pain signals from reaching the brain. And second, when the acupuncture needles are pushed into the skin they also stimulate the production of the endorphins, the body's own pain-relieving hormones. Together these changes ensure that the patient will gradually become less and less aware of the pain about which he has previously complained.

In addition to providing us with this explanation as to how acupuncture works, scientists have also produced evidence which shows that it is not necessary to follow the traditional acupuncture meridians in order to obtain this effect. It is, in fact, possible to obtain exactly the same effect by stimulating any point on a fairly large area of skin.

Finally, and perhaps most dramatically of all, scientists

have shown that it is possible to obtain this same acupuncture effect without sticking needles into the skin at all! It is, it seems, perfectly possible to close the spinal cord gate and stimulate the production of endorphins by applying heat or electrical stimulation to the body, or even by applying finger pressure to tender pressure points.

And that is where modern research takes us full circle, for there is another ancient Chinese form of medical practice called *shiatsu* in which pain is relieved simply by pressing on the skin.

Hypnotherapy

Hypnotherapy fascinated the Egyptians several thousand years ago, and in the seventeenth century a microscopist called Athanasius Kircher played around with the idea, but it wasn't until Franz Mesmer developed the concept in the late eighteenth century that hypnosis and hypnotherapy really came of age.

The first evidence that hypnotherapy can help patients in pain came in 1847, when a surgeon called James Esdale reported that he had performed 300 major surgical operations in India using hypnosis as the only anaesthetic. His report, and others like it, might have attracted more attention had not the nineteenth century also seen the development of gas anaesthesia and drugs such as aspirin. As it was, hypnosis drifted into a quiet medical backwater.

During the last couple of decades, however, hypnosis has come back into fashion once again, and numerous people now claim that hypnotherapy is an excellent way of dealing with pain. Once again major surgery has been done on hypnotized patients, and in one remarkable experiment conducted recently it was shown that hypnosis can be more effective than morphine as a pain reliever. Studies have demonstrated that hypnosis raises both pain threshold and pain tolerance levels.

Popular though hypnotherapy has now become it does, however, seem clear that it is not necessary to visit a hypnotist in order to benefit from the quality of pain relief associated with this alternative branch of medicine. It is, apparently, perfectly possible to obtain all the benefits associated with hypnotherapy through self-hypnosis. Indeed, the patient who learns how to use self-hypnosis properly will have two important advantages over the patient who is dependent on a professional hypnotherapist: the benefits will be easier to obtain, and they will last longer too.

Conclusions

There are numerous useful alternative medical specialities. And there is little doubt that patients in pain can benefit from many of these techniques. Acupuncture and hypnotherapy are just two of the useful specialities that have become popular in recent years.

Until now, however, patients wanting to try alternative medical specialities have faced a number of problems. The first and most significant has been the difficulty of identifying a safe and responsible practitioner of alternative medicine. There are some good, honest, reliable alternative practitioners around. But, unfortunately, there are many quacks and charlatans who have obtained their mail-order diplomas after a few hours' postal tuition and whose knowledge of human biology and behaviour would not entitle them to a simple 'O' level general science pass.

Sadly, many patients have been misled, misinformed and cheated of large amounts of money by dishonest acupuncturists and hypnotherapists. Many more have suffered serious injury at the hands of unskilled and careless practitioners. Unfortunately, it is difficult if not impossible for the ordinary patient to differentiate between the honest and honourable and the dishonest and dishonourable.

Happily, however, there is now an overwhelming amount of evidence to show that any of these really useful benefits that can be obtained by visiting alternative practitioners can be obtained at home without cost, risk or inconvenience.

PART THREE

The Pain Control Programme

Introduction

Pain isn't just a natural response to a threat or injury; it's much more than that. As I explained earlier in this book (on pages 29–40) pain is influenced by an extraordinary number of different factors. Anxiety, depression and fear can all make it worse, and the psychological factors which lead to the development of a pain are often far more significant than the purely physical factors.

This does not mean that the pain isn't real, or that the patient is 'malingering' or 'putting it on'; far from it, a pain for which there is no obvious physical explanation can be just as cruelly terrifying, just as debilitating and just as tiring as a pain for which there is an immediate and obvious explanation.

In just the same way that pain is often produced by indefinable factors and influences, so it can often also be controlled by powers and techniques which may at first be difficult to understand. The Pain Control Programme that follows is specially designed to take full advantage of the many ways in which you can use your own body and mind to help combat pain.

Before you study my Pain Control Programme there are one or two important points I must make.

First, the techniques I have described here are designed to help you control recurrent or persistent pain rather than sudden, acute or emergency pain. If your pain has lasted for more than a month or so and your doctors are unable to provide you with a solution, then my Pain Control Programme will certainly help you.

Second, you must, of course, continue any treatment that you are already receiving from your doctor. The techniques described on the pages which follow will not interfere with any other treatment you may need. The only thing to remember is that by using these techniques your need for medication or other medical aids may be reduced.

Third, if your condition changes in any way, or if you develop an acute pain of any kind, then you must always contact your own doctor first. Do not attempt to deal with any new or unexplained pain with any of the techniques described in my Pain Control Programme. If you do, there is a real danger that you will 'mask' important symptoms which might help your doctor produce a precise diagnosis.

Fourth, remember that even though it is not always possible to *abolish* pain completely it is invariably possible to *reduce* pain to bearable levels. I don't promise that my Programme will banish your pains. But I do promise that, if you follow my instructions carefully, your pain will be reduced.

Fifth, my Pain Control Programme consists of a number of different techniques and approaches. You should try them all. Some may not work for you. Some may seem especially appropriate. But it is important to remember that when put together these techniques will help you far more than they would if operated in isolation. The more aspects of my Pain Control Programme that you can employ, the greater will be the amount of pain relief you enjoy.

Sixth, try to suspend your natural sense of scepticism. If you have received any sort of scientific training then you will have almost certainly been taught to believe that pain can only be controlled by drugs or surgery. That theory is as outdated as the theory of 'specificity'. The gate control theory showed that pain control can be achieved by the enhancement of normal, physiological activities. It also showed that the disruption or masking of sensory impulses by destructive, irreversible surgical lesions, or by the over-zealous use of drugs, is not good medical practice. As you read through the pages which follow you should remember that since we know now that the human mind can both produce pain and make existing pain worse, it is undeniably possible that the human mind can eradicate or control that very same pain.

Finally, before you start studying my Pain Control Programme, decide exactly what your goals are. Do you want to be able to sleep at night? Do you want to be able to move around a little more freely? Do you want to be able to start work again? Do you want to be able to cut down your dependence on drugs?

If you can define your goals you are far more likely to be able to achieve them.

Know Your Illness

If you're worried about what is causing your pain, or you don't understand what is wrong with you, then your pain will be made much worse than it need be.

Imagine, for example, that you've banged your head and acquired a headache. When you get home you look in the bathroom mirror and notice that you have a graze on your forehead and the beginnings of what will undoubtedly turn out to be a fairly large bruise.

You may need to sit down and take things easy for a while, you may even need to take a couple of aspirin tablets. But you won't worry much about the headache. You'll know what caused it and you'll know that it will disappear fairly quickly. Within a few hours the headache will have probably gone completely. All you'll have left to remind you of your accident will be a bruise.

Now, imagine that on your way home after banging your head you met a well-meaning friend who, when he hears that you have a headache, tells you that he once heard of someone who developed severe internal bleeding after a headache and ended up paralysed for many months.

This time when you get home you won't be quite so calm about your headache. You'll begin to worry about it. You'll wonder whether or not you could be bleeding internally. You'll wonder whether or not you're likely to end up paralysed.

Within an hour or two you may well be worrying about what will happen to your job while you are struggling to recover. You'll worry about how the mortgage will get paid. You'll worry about your relatives and your dependants. And you'll continually examine your arms and legs to see if there is any sign of developing weakness or paralysis.

Your anxieties and your fears will make your muscles so tense that after a few hours your headache will be getting worse, not better. You won't be able to relax or rest. You'll be convinced that something terrible is about to happen. Your headache will get so bad that you have to go to bed and lie down.

But just before you bury yourself underneath the sheets you'll probably make one last desperate telephone call: you'll telephone your doctor and ask him to come and see you.

When your doctor arrives he'll examine you carefully and after about five minutes probably tell you that he can't find anything at all for you to worry about. You have a small bruise developing but there are no signs that you have damaged yourself in any other way. Relieved, you thank him, get up and make a cup of tea.

Within ten minutes you will have relaxed so much that your tension will have virtually disappeared.

And your headache will have gone too.

A few years ago doctors believed that patients were better off if they didn't know anything about their illness or the treatment they required. There are, I suspect, still quite a few doctors around who still believe that. But there is now a tremendous amount of evidence to show that the opposite is true: most patients are much less likely to suffer unnecessary pain if they are told what is wrong with them, warned what to expect, and given advice on exactly how to cope with their problems.

There have been several specific research projects which have proved this point. In one study, for example, ninety-seven patients who were in hospital to have surgical operations were told exactly what to expect and what sort of pain they would have to put up with after their operations. Indeed, the patients weren't just told what sort of pain to expect; they were also told how they could most effectively deal with the pain that they developed. They were taught how to relax their muscles, they were told to breathe deeply but slowly, and they were told how to move around so that they put the least amount of strain on their wounds.

After they had their operations these ninety-seven patients needed half the amount of pain-killing medication required by a control group of patients who had been given no specific instructions, and who had not been told what to expect. In addition the patients who had been given instructions were, on average, ready to go home three days earlier than the patients who'd not been told what sort of pains to expect.

Similar results have been obtained whenever this type of study has been repeated. It doesn't matter what sort of operation the patients need: they suffer less pain if they are told what to expect. And, of course, this isn't just true of patients needing surgical operations. It just happens to be easier to prove the point with patients who are having surgery, since with such patients it is fairly easy to define just when their pain should start.

Whatever your illness may be, you will suffer far less pain if you find out as much about it as you possibly can.

Pain Control Programme prescription

I suggest that you try to follow these instructions as carefully and as conscientiously as you can.

1. If you are in any doubt about what is causing your pain ask your doctor to tell you everything he knows about your problem. If your doctor cannot explain things to you satisfactorily, ask your doctor to arrange for you to see a hospital specialist. Then ask the specialist to tell you as much as he can about your condition. If you still don't understand what is happening, ask for details of the diagnosis that has been made and look up your disease in a book in your local library. Read as much as you possibly can about your problem. If your disorder is a common one then there will probably be books in your local bookshop which will explain your condition comprehensively. If your condition is less well known then you may need to study a medical textbook with

a dictionary by your elbow. Don't let yourself be put off by medical jargon.

It is natural to worry about your health if you're in constant pain. The more you know about the cause of your pain, and the more you understand what is going on, the less you'll worry. And the less pain you'll suffer.

2. Remember that in the majority of cases recurrent or persistent pain cannot be explained. It is very likely that your doctors will not be able to give you a specific explanation for your pain for the very simple reason that they have not been able to make a diagnosis or find anything physically wrong with you.

Do not allow yourself to be disheartened by this.

It is perfectly possible to suffer severe, persistent or recurrent pain without there being anything physically wrong. This does not mean that you are imagining your pain. But it does mean that you probably don't have to worry about your future health. You can concentrate on battling against your pain – which is an end in itself and not a sign of some underlying abnormality.

3. Whether your doctors have produced a diagnosis or not, try to decide what activities make your pains worse and what activities seem to make it better. And then try to find ways of avoiding the activities which produce pain and of increasing your participation in activities which reduce pain. If sitting in an easy chair always makes your pain worse then don't sit in easy chairs. Don't try forcing yourself to do things which are painful.

Use Drugs Wisely

Drugs often play a vital part in controlling pain. But they are often abused and over-used, with the result that the side effects and complications they produce exceed the advantages they offer. Even drugs as simple as aspirin can have a profound effect on your body and your mind; they can cause an enormous range of disturbing and damaging problems. Under some circumstances patients suffering from persistent or recurrent pain can even become addicted to the drugs they are taking (although I do stress that this doesn't happen when powerful drugs such as morphine are used simply to help control very severe pain).

Pain Control Programme prescription

Try to follow these instructions as carefully and as conscientiously as you can.

1. Remember that drugs should only ever play a *part* in your personal Pain Control Programme. Drugs can often help relieve pain. But they are not the only answer.

2. If you are taking drugs regularly you should take them at fixed times. You should not wait until your pain returns. If you only take drugs when you have a pain you will eventually become addicted to your drugs. If you are receiving pain-killing injections persuade your doctor or nurse to give you your injections at regular intervals and *not* when the pain has returned.

3. Do not take more than one lot of drugs at once unless your doctor has specifically instructed you to do so. Drugs do not mix well, and if you take a drug that you have bought from your local chemist's at the same time as you are taking a drug that your doctor has prescribed then there may well be an unpleasant and unexpected interaction.

4. Do not take a tranquillizing drug to help relieve pain. The most commonly prescribed tranquillizers, the benzodiazepines such as Valium, Librium, Mogadon and Ativan, are unlikely to help relieve your pain and may indeed make it worse. These drugs are at least as addictive as heroin and do not have any specific pain-killing qualities. They will make you drowsy and numb your reactions, and reduce your chances of successfully defeating your pain.

5. If you want to cut down your consumption of drugs, cut down the dosage you take rather than the number of times you take the drug. So, for example, if you take three aspirin tablets four times a day then cut down to two tablets four times a day rather than taking three tablets three times a day. As a general rule you should try to ensure that you take the smallest drug dose possible.

6. If you notice any side effects or unexpected symptoms while taking a drug, you should assume that the new symptoms are caused by the drug you are taking. You should speak to your doctor straight away and ask his advice.

7. Remember that drugs can only ever mask a condition, they cannot cure it. No pill, however powerful, can provide a permanent solution to your pain.

Use Your Imagination

If you've ever watched a television film taken by a camera fitted inside a roller coaster car then you'll know how easily your mind can be misled and how your senses can fool your imagination. As the roller coaster climbs and dives you can feel your stomach churning and your last meal struggling to escape even though you're still sitting comfortably in your living-room chair. Your body responds not to reality but to what it thinks is happening.

Doctors and psychologists have been aware of this phenomenon for some time. When the film *Lawrence of Arabia* was shown on cinema screens a few years ago the sales of ice cream and cold drinks rocketed: the patrons watching the hot desert scenes all felt hot and needed to cool off by eating or drinking something chilly.

This doesn't only happen when you have a television or cinema picture to stimulate your mind.

Most of us are constantly creating images and scenarios for ourselves simply by thinking about things. Invariably we then respond to our created images and scenarios.

If you are worried that you are going to be made redundant, your body will respond to your fears: your heart will beat faster, your blood pressure will go up and your muscles will become tense. You'll develop a headache, not because you have been made redundant but because you have been thinking about being made redundant. If you think that your mild stomach pains could be caused by cancer then your pains will get much worse. If a young girl thinks that her periods are always going to be painful then she'll tense her muscles as each period approaches.

Exactly how the imagination manages to exert this quite

remarkable power over the body is still something of a mystery. But to a large extent the 'how' is purely academic. The indisputable fact is that even though we may not know exactly how it works the human mind will respond to scenes it has imagined just as positively and dramatically as it will respond to reality.

Until fairly recently most of the evidence linking the human imagination to pain was evidence which showed that by thinking about unhappy, miserable things you could make yourself ill or create new pains for yourself. But in the last few years there have been a number of experiments which have shown, quite conclusively, that the human imagination can also have a very dramatic positive effect. By learning to use your imagination you can get rid of pain.

The first major experiment I've been able to find which tested the ability of the imagination to have a useful effect on the body's perception of pain was conducted by John Horan and John Dellinger of Pennsylvania State University and published in an American journal, *Perceptual and Motor Skills*, in 1974.

Horan and Dellinger conducted their experiment in two parts. In the first experiment their thirty-six volunteer subjects were instructed to place their right hands in ice water and to hold their hands in the water for as long as they possibly could. If you've ever dipped your hands into a bucket of icy water then you'll know that it isn't just an unpleasant experience; after a few seconds it becomes positively painful. The human hand doesn't *like* being held in icy water and it quickly tells the brain that it is in pain.

In the second experiment Horan and Dellinger asked their volunteers to keep their hands in ice water again, but this time they told them to try and imagine pleasant scenes. They were told to try to imagine that instead of sitting in a laboratory with one hand in freezing cold water they were walking through a lush green meadow or sitting looking at a beautiful blue lake. The results were quite remarkable.

In the first experiment the men in the group managed to keep their hands in the ice water for an average of 69 seconds. The women managed to keep their hands in the ice water for a mere 34 seconds.

In the second experiment, however, when they were encouraged to use their imaginations to help them keep their hands in the ice water for as long as possible, the men managed an average of 117 seconds while the women managed an average of 176 seconds. As so many other experiments were to confirm in subsequent years, women tend to respond much more readily to their imaginations than do men – perhaps because they are less likely to be resistant to the idea, less likely to have a strictly scientific background and less likely to think the whole concept silly or preposterous.

With fairly minor variations this experiment was conducted many more times in the following few years.

In 1977, for example, Donald Scott and Theodore Barber, both from Medfield in Massachusetts, reported that they had conducted an experiment using eighty undergraduates from a college in Boston.

Their eighty volunteers were each paid three dollars to stick their hands in icy water but, because it had been shown that most people can keep their dominant hand in cold water for a slightly longer time than they can keep their non-dominant hand in cold water, Scott and Barber told their volunteer subjects to stick their dominant hands in the ice bucket. The right-handed individuals stuck their right hands in the bucket; the left-handed subjects stuck their left hands in the water. Once again the experiment was conducted in two stages.

In the first stage members of a control group were told simply to keep their hands in the ice water for as long as possible.

In the second part of the experiment the students were told: 'There are two ways that you can react to this test. One way is to get all fussed up and bothered about the sensations. The other way is to use some strategies that will affect your perception of pain and your ability to tolerate it. One strategy you can use while your hand is in the apparatus is to concentrate on other things all during this time. Another strategy you can use is to become aware of the sensations, but do not think of them as painful, but as unusual sensations. A related way is to think of your hand as a wax or rubber hand and not really part of you. A final strategy you can use when the sensations level off is to think as if your hand feels dull and insensitive.'

Once again the results were extremely convincing. The volunteers who were merely told to try and hold their hands in icy water for as long as possible managed an average of 279 seconds while the volunteers who were given the alternative strategies for dealing with their pain managed an average of 435 seconds. (Since they managed to keep their hands in the icy water for much longer even as controls, it seems fair to assume either that this group of volunteers was much hardier than the group used by Scott and Barber or that the water wasn't quite as cold.)

A year later, in 1978, Matt Jaremko of the University of Richmond in Virginia conducted another experiment which proved the same point. Jaremko told his volunteers to imagine that they were in a desert on a hot day and that they were feeling uncomfortably tired. He told them to think of the ice water into which they were plunging their hands as cool and refreshing. Jaremko concluded that the technique worked remarkably well but added that 'The extent to which a person gets involved with imagining the strategies has an influence on the effect of changing pain tolerance. Those who are highly involved show a pronounced enhancement effect.'

During the last few years more evidence to support the theory that the imagination can influence the body's ability to cope with pain has come in thick and fast. Dr Lorne Hartman, Director of the Behavior Therapy Program at the Clarke Institute of Psychiatry in Toronto, and Kenneth Ainsworth, Psychometrist in the Department of Psychology at Chedoke Hospital in Hamilton, Ontario, published a report in the *Canadian Journal of Psychiatry* in 1980 which showed that by using their imagination to picture gentle, peaceful images patients could successfully control their pain. Michael Rosenbaum of Haifa University in Israel has recently obtained similar results.

I've described a number of the research projects which show that pain can be controlled by using the imagination simply because I suspect that many people will find the whole concept difficult to accept. Most of us have been brought up in a world where the unexplained and the inexplicable are, often rightly, regarded with suspicion. Anyone who has any sort of scientific training will have been taught to regard with suspicion any claim that 'hidden mental powers' can be used to combat genuine physical illness.

And yet, as the research papers which I've quoted show quite conclusively, we *can* use our imagination to help us control pain. Our imagination can produce problems and create pain, but it can also solve problems and eradicate pain. It may sound unlikely, but the evidence proves that if you imagine a situation which is inconsistent with pain, and if your imagery is convincing, then you will suffer less pain.

Pain Control Programme prescription

You can use your imagination to help control your pain in a number of quite different ways, but there are two basic approaches which you can follow.

First, you can use your imagination to create pleasant and relaxing scenes. If you imagine that you are sitting on a grassy bank overlooking a beautiful lake and that you can see a heron, a kingfisher and all sorts of other beautiful birds around you, the chances are that any pain you are feeling will be reduced in quantity and quality.

Second, you can use your imagination in a much more aggressive way. In one recent experiment, for example, patients were asked to concentrate on the parts of their bodies where their pains were most intense. They were then asked to visualize the shape of their pain and to imagine that their pain had a vivid red line all the way around its boundary.

Having done that the patients were asked to watch their pain slowly getting smaller and smaller. After the patients had done this for fifteen to twenty minutes the researchers found that the intensity of the pain fell at about the same rate as the size of the area of pain was reduced.

Today this type of aggressive technique is being used more and more frequently – and with astonishingly successful results.

It really doesn't matter all that much which approach you use – both will help you. But the important thing to remember is that you will benefit most from this pain-controlling technique if you create your own images. Read through the techniques I describe on the following pages, and then use my examples to help you create your own pain-controlling images. You will find that your body responds most dramatically to those images which you yourself have developed. In addition you will find that you benefit enormously from the feeling that your pain is under your *own* personal control.

The passive imagery techniques are similar to the techniques which were used in the experiments which originally proved the value of the power of the human imagination in dealing with pain. You should remember that these techniques are designed to be used in short bursts. You should 'disappear' into your imaginary world only when your pain is particularly troublesome or is interfering with some other activity (such as trying to get to sleep).

You should, of course, also remember that you will not benefit from these techniques unless you are prepared to spend some time practising. If you wanted to learn to play golf then you wouldn't expect to be able to master the game after one fifteen-minute session. If you wanted to learn how to dance the tango you wouldn't expect to be proficient after one dance. Similarly, you shouldn't expect to be able to conquer your pain completely at your first attempt. You must be prepared to spend fifteen or twenty minutes a day practising, every day for a week. And, ideally, you should practice your skills when your pain is at its weakest. You will undoubtedly gain some benefit on your first attempt – the experiments which I have quoted above were, after all, conducted without any practice or rehearsals – but you will not obtain the full benefit from this aspect of the Pain Control Programme unless you are prepared to spend some time practising.

Here are a few simple 'daydreams' for you to try. Remember that I offer these only as samples. By using your own memory and imagination you should be able to create scenes of your own.

1. Imagine that you are walking along a pleasant country lane in early summer. The narrow lane is quite deserted and you are completely alone. On either side of you the hedgerows are overgrown and full of colourful wild flowers. On the other side of the hedges there are meadows of wonderful green grass, decorated only with dancing red poppies and dazzling yellow buttercups.

As you walk along the lane you can hear dozens of different birds busily singing. There are sparrows, wrens, blue tits, blackbirds and thrushes. Every so often there is an oak tree standing in the hedgerow and each time you come to a tree you stand for a few moments relaxing in the shade that the tree provides. On one such occasion you casually glance over the top of the hedge and find yourself watching a hare playing just a few feet inside the meadow. He seems oblivious to your presence and you watch him for several minutes.

When you started your walk the lane seemed to stretch into the distance. You could see no sign of it ending. Now you notice that the lane is about to fall down into a pleasant, lightly wooded valley. Just before the lane starts to fall away there is a narrow stone bridge and underneath the bridge a clear stream splashes its way across a mass of water-smoothed pebbles and rocks.

You stop for a moment, see that there is a narrow path leading down to the stream and clamber down until you are standing on the bank. The grass here is particularly green and soft; it is mixed with clover and has a wonderfully springy texture to it. You look around, find a spot where you can sit with your back leaning against a tree and settle down with the stream busily chattering away to itself no more than a foot from your feet. In the water you can see a small river trout looking for food. On the other side of the bank a kingfisher sits, waiting to pounce. And a little further up the stream you hear a slight splash as an otter dives into a deeper part of the stream.

2. Imagine that you are sitting in your bedroom in a large, comfortable and rather expensive country hotel. The cost of the room doesn't concern you in the slightest. You have no worries about money. You are wearing nothing but a dressing gown which is tied loosely around your waist. You are sitting in a leather armchair and watching a crackling log fire. Occasionally you have to move forward to throw another log onto the fire.

Behind you there is a four-poster bed that is hung with a brocade canopy made of a rich red and gold material. Matching curtains hang at all four corners of the bed and are tied back with red ropes, fastened neatly in bows.

The room is panelled in oak and there is one window on your right. It is an old-fashioned diamond-paned leaded window with thick, red velvet curtains hanging on each side of it. If you turned your head to the right you would be able to look through the window at a corner of a beautiful, peaceful, typically English garden. Beyond, in the distance, you'd be able to see countless acres of rolling countryside. In front of the window there is a long window seat covered in material that matches the curtains.

The door to the room is on your left and almost impossible to distinguish from the walls. It is made of exactly the same sort of oak as the panelling. A large, old-fashioned key protrudes from the lock and the bolt has been drawn as an added security.

Outside the weather is freezing cold, but in your bedroom the temperature is comfortably warm. You spent the morning walking across the hills and you can still remember the bite of the cool winter air. The mud tracks in the rough lane leading to the hotel were frozen solid.

You had lunch in a traditional old-fashioned public house a few miles away from the hotel and arrived back at the hotel an hour or so ago. You had a piping-hot bath in an old-fashioned bathroom with an extraordinarily large bath in it. After you'd finished your bath you asked the hotel reception to send up a tray of tea and muffins.

As you sit watching the fire you smile contentedly. Life is really very good for you.

3. You are on the Orient-Express heading for Venice. You have a compartment of your own and for the next twenty-four hours you have absolutely nothing to worry about.

An hour or so ago you finished lunch and three other passengers invited you to join them for liqueurs and a game of cards in the lounge. They are an interesting-looking trio.

You said that you'd be delighted and agreed to meet them again in the lounge in half an hour or so. At the moment you're resting in your compartment, watching the scenery flash past and enjoying the unashamed luxury of the compartment's expensive fittings.

Luncheon was quite spectacular. You've never eaten nor drunk so well in your life. The service was excellent. And there was something undeniably exciting about enjoying a meal on the train that has starred in so many books and films.

Suddenly your mind flashes back to Paris. You've just spent three weeks there at a splendid hotel right in the heart of the city. You spent your final evening having dinner at Maxim's and wandering up and down the Champs-Elysées with an American friend you met at the hotel. You're on your way to spend ten days in Venice and then you'll be going back to Paris. You've promised to meet your American friend again on your first evening back in the French capital. You've got a table booked at Maxim's.

The combination of the wine you had at lunch and the gentle motion of the train is threatening to send you to sleep. Outside it is just beginning to snow again and you suspect that within an hour or two the fields through which your train is passing will be carpeted in snow. You're glad you brought a warm fur coat with you even though it is wonderfully warm in your compartment. You know that at this time of year Venice can sometimes be rather chilly.

You look at your watch. You've still got twenty minutes before you're due to meet your travelling companions. You decide that you'll just lie down for a while and have a snooze.

4. Imagine that you're lying on a warm, sunny beach. It is a day in midsummer and yet the beach is quite deserted. In the distance to your right and to your left there are one or

two families scattered around, and you can hear the sound of children playing. But there isn't anyone close to you and the noises are very distant. In front of you the waves are breaking gently on the soft sand and behind you a slight breeze rustles through the long grasses growing in the sand dunes.

High, high above you you can hear the seagulls calling to one another as they circle overhead. They and the distant children are the only sounds that disturb the peace and tranquillity of the afternoon.

The most insistent sensation is that of warmth. The sand underneath you is warm and the sun is warm on your skin. You have oiled yourself carefully with sun lotion and you can smell it still. If you opened your eyes you'd be able to see your skin glistening in the sunshine. But the sun is bright on your eyelids and you don't want to open your eyes just yet.

You lie there, quite still and peaceful, soaking up the sun and enjoying the afternoon warmth.

To begin with, practise these daydreams somewhere comfortable where you can lie down. Your bedroom is probably the best place. Close the door and lock it if you can. Put a 'Do Not Disturb' notice on the outside door handle. Lie yourself down on your bed and make yourself as comfortable as you can.

Read through one of these scenes slowly and try to see yourself in the situations I have described. Alternatively you can ask someone close to you to read the words out slowly and softly while you are lying down and feeling comfortably relaxed.

As the weeks go by you can build up a library of your own favourite, private daydreams. Some of them can be real, some may be based on memories taken from films, television programmes or books and others may be purely imaginary. It really doesn't matter where you get your daydreams from as long as your mind can believe them.

You can use these daydreams to relax your mind and help control your pain whenever you feel tension building up inside you, or whenever your pain is difficult to bear.

Most of the early research that was done to show that the power of the imagination could be used to help combat pain was done with the aid of simple, passive techniques such as the ones I have described above. The volunteers were asked to imagine that they were enjoying a pleasant or relaxing scene, or to see themselves resting in beautiful surroundings.

More recently, however, it has been shown that the imagination can be used in a much more constructive way to help patients conquer pain. By regarding your pain as an enemy and by developing a range of imaginative combative skills you can take a much more active part in the control of your pain.

To give you an idea of some of the ways that you can use your imagination in a positive and combative way I have listed below some simple introductory techniques that are well worth trying. Do remember, however, that as with passive imaginative techniques you will benefit most if you develop and use your own images.

1. Imagine that your pain is being transmitted around your body via a series of thin wires. Try to see wires connecting your brain to every single part of your body that hurts. Now, imagine that deep inside your body there is a small fighting force of miniature physicians. Each physician is equipped with a strong pair of wire cutters. One by one your tiny physicians cut your pain-transmitting wires. As each wire is cut, you suddenly realize that the amount of pain you feel in that area is quite dramatically reduced.

2. Imagine that you can see the pain in your body as a small invading army of dirty brown cells. Imagine that every pain sensation in your body is produced by one of these cells. Now imagine that your body's own fighting forces, your white cells, are regrouping to attack the invaders. Imagine that your white cells have been quietly building up their forces for several hours and that they are ready to tackle the pain producers.

Next, imagine that the white cells are fighting and destroying the dirty, brown invading cells. Imagine that the brown cells are littering your tissues with their rapidly decaying corpses.

Your white cells, your personal fighting force, are winning their battle.

3. Imagine that you have left your body and that you are watching yourself from the other side of the room. Imagine that as you watch a pretty young nurse approaches and soothes your body. Imagine that there are loving, compassionate, ever gentle people around you and helping to ease your pain. When the pain has been banished from your body then you can return to it.

4. Another technique is to try and alter the context in which your pain has appeared. If you're sitting in the dentist's chair and waiting for him to attack your teeth with his drill then imagine that your dentist is a ruthless police interrogator and that you are a spy desperately trying hard to protect your sources and your companions. Imagine that every move the dentist makes is designed to help him gouge information out of you. And imagine that you are equally determined to ensure that he does not succeed.

Or there is another one that you could try if you have legs that are arthritic and painful to move. Imagine that you are a fighter pilot and that you've parachuted out over enemy country. Imagine that you injured your legs when you baled out of your aeroplane. Imagine that you need to regain the full use of your legs as soon as possible so that you can get back through enemy lines with the valuable information that you've obtained.

These scenarios may sound extreme and even slightly odd. You may not expect a doctor to suggest that you conquer your pain by losing yourself in a Walter Mitty type fantasy.

But in both these instances, by creating an acceptable imaginary situation for your pain you will increase your pain tolerance level noticeably. Your mind will accept your pain as a problem that must be overcome.

5. Try using your imagination and the creative part of your brain in harness. Try devising limericks or songs. Try

remembering all the names of the friends you had when you were twelve years old. Try doing mathematics problems in your head. Try working out chess problems without a board. Imagine that you have to write an article about your pain or that you have to plan a lecture describing the ways in which pain can affect an individual's life. It really doesn't matter *what* you do; the important thing is that you find something that you are interested in and that you can be enthusiastic about.

6. I hardly dare mention this because I suspect that it will offend some people, but I do think it's important so if you are easily offended then please skip the next few lines!

Try thinking of something sexy. For many people there is nothing more invigorating or exciting than escapist sexual fantasy. Black stockings, suspenders, bondage, troilism – it really doesn't matter what you fantasize about as long as your imagination is powerful enough to create a believable fantasy. There are dozens of magazines now available for people who want to develop their skills as sexual fantasists but who aren't quite sure how to go about it.

Learn to Laugh

I don't think anyone really knows exactly why laughter and humour have such a positive pain-relieving effect. And there isn't yet any solid research evidence to prove that by laughing you can reduce the amount of pain in your life. But the amount of reliable anecdotal evidence is convincing.

One of the best-known patients to defeat pain with the therapeutic benefits of laughter was the American magazine editor Norman Cousins. Mr Cousins described his personal experiences in his book *The Anatomy of an Illness*, and a film starring Ed Asner as Norman Cousins was later made, based on the book.

Having been diagnosed as suffering from ankylosing spondylitis, a crippling inflammatory disease for which there is no known cure, Norman Cousins was told by his doctors that there was nothing they could do for him apart from prescribe pain killers.

Desperately unhappy about his condition, Cousins refused to lie back and just take his medicine. He decided to try and cheer himself up by making a deliberate attempt to make himself laugh. He hired a projector and some of his favourite comedy films, and he started rereading books by some of his favourite humorous writers.

When the hospital staff complained that all the laughter coming from his room was disturbing the other patients, Cousins moved out of the hospital and into a room in a hotel across the street. There he continued with his unusual regimen of daily laughter.

The experiment was a tremendous success. Several extremely eminent physicians had forecast that Cousins would never be able to move freely again, but within months he was walking, swimming and back at his old job again. Just as important in scientific terms was the fact that with the aid of his doctor Cousins managed to show that his laughter had a useful, positive, practical effect on his physical condition.

The hospital laboratory showed that by laughing Cousins had succeeded in reducing the amount of inflammatory change in his body. He had actually managed to laugh himself better.

As I have already said, scientists still don't know why laughter has such a useful effect. It has been suggested that laughter may help by improving respiration, by lowering blood pressure and, possibly, by increasing the supply of specific types of internally produced hormones. It may be that laughter works by diverting attention away from the pain. It may be, as Dr Paul Ekman of the University of California has claimed, that the very act of flexing the facial muscles into a smile may produce a genuine and calming effect on the nervous system, heart rate and respiratory system. (Don't dismiss this theory: next time you're feeling miserable or in pain try putting a really cheerful smile on to your face. You'll find that it really does help. Try making your eyes sparkle with laughter and you'll notice the effect even more.)

We are going to have to wait for scientists to do more research before we know exactly how laughter can have such a positive effect on pain. But meanwhile it seems silly not to take full advantage of the fact that laughter is an effective therapy; it does help eradicate pain.

And it has several other advantages too: it doesn't cost anything, and there aren't any side effects.

Pain Control Programme prescription

1. Make a list of your favourite funny films and books. If you have a video recorder try to keep copies of films that you find particularly pleasing – and that you know you can rely on to provide you with an hour or two of genuine

amusement. Try to find films that actually make you laugh out loud.

And keep a library of your favourite funny books too. It's impossible for me to recommend books because your taste in humour may not be the same as mine. But the number of humour books published today is so huge that you're bound to be able to find several to your own particular taste. If you want to try classic 'funny' authors try Jerome K. Jerome, James Thurber, Stephen Leacock, Robert Benchley and S. J. Perelman. You can always ask your local librarian to recommend authors to you.

2. Try to spend as much time as possible with people who are generally happy and cheerful rather than sad and miserable.

If you spend your days with people who always have long faces and always look on the black side, the chances are that eventually you will acquire a long face and a gloomy view of life. Depression is contagious. Bright and cheerful friends will probably do you far more good than any pain-killing pills your doctor can prescribe.

3. Do try not to take yourself – or life – too seriously. Many people with reasonably responsible jobs feel that they have to maintain a serious demeanour at all times. They're quite wrong. As long as you take care to preserve your serious manner for the times when it really matters, you'll lose absolutely nothing by allowing yourself to laugh occasionally.

And do remember that it isn't always the expensive things in life which provide the most pleasure. When did you last buy a copy of a children's comic – one of the comics you used to enjoy so much when you were small, for example? When did you last visit a joke shop? When did you last buy a book of cartoons? When did you last find the time to stop and watch children playing in the park or young folk messing about in boats on the river?

4. If you are a naturally pessimistic individual, try to suppress your pessimism and replace it with optimism. Try to start each day in as cheerful and optimistic a frame of

mind as possible. If you get up in the morning thinking of all the terrible chores that you've got to do, and thinking constantly about how much your pain is ruining your life, it won't take much else to turn a potentially bad day into a truly awful experience. If something goes wrong early on in the day then your attitude will simply make things worse. As you go through the day with your scowl and your gloomy demeanour the people you meet will be depressed by your approach. It won't be surprising if they respond accordingly. And by evening you'll be in a deep, dark depression. Your pessimism will have rebounded on you and rebuilt your own fear and misery. Your depression, confusion, fear, anger and consequent frustration will together all help make your pain worse.

I know that if your pain is troublesome or ever threatening it isn't always easy to be optimistic. But it is important to try. Instead of thinking in negative terms, try to think of all the positive, encouraging aspects of your life.

Think of the things in your life which are enjoyable. Think of the events that you can look forward to. And try to take as much pleasure as possible from every enjoyable experience you have.

5. If you find that it is impossible to think in optimistic terms, or if you find it impossible to laugh, then you should consult your doctor and explain to him how you feel. Depression and pain often go together in a vicious and debilitating circle. Pain produces depression and depression makes pain worse. It can be difficult to break out of the cycle, but your doctor can today often prescribe useful and effective anti-depressant drugs.

Getting to Sleep

Patients who suffer from pain frequently have difficulty in getting to sleep at night. It's not difficult to understand why this happens, of course. Anyone who has ever suffered from pain will confirm that it is difficult if not impossible to get a good night's sleep for as long as the pain persists. The whole problem is made much worse by the fact that patients who suffer from persistent pain tend to suffer more in the late evening. According to a study conducted by anaesthetists in both Australia and Great Britain, patients who suffer from chronic pain tend to be at their worst at about ten o'clock in the evening. Anxiety and depression also tend to get much worse at about this time too.

Since it is when we are asleep that we recharge our personal batteries, getting a good night's sleep is vitally important. Any patient whose ability to sleep at night is impaired should read the following section very carefully.

Pain Control Programme prescription

1. Pain killers are the only pills that you should take to help you get to sleep. And as I have explained elsewhere in this book (on page 55) the only two drugs worth using are aspirin and morphine.

Many hundreds of thousands of patients who suffer from persistent pain take sleeping tablets at night. I don't think this is a very good idea.

The main reason for my disapproval is that the most commonly prescribed sleeping tablets are drugs in the benzodiazepine group of tranquillizers. Not only do these drugs cause a wide range of unfortunate physical side effects but they also have three quite specific and damaging effects which are likely to have an adverse effect on any patient suffering from pain.

First, most of the benzodiazepine sleeping tablets have an effect which lasts much longer than a single night. This means that a patient who takes a tranquillizing sleeping tablet at ten o'clock one evening will still be 'tranquillized' throughout the following day. The inevitable result of this is that he or she will find it difficult to concentrate and dangerous to move about. The tablet the pain sufferer takes to help him get a night's sleep will turn him into a permanent invalid.

Second, and even more important, most of the benzodiazepine sleeping tablets are designed for a very short-term use only. If pills of this type are taken for more than a couple of weeks they start to cause insomnia. The patient, not realizing what is happening, will probably increase his nighttime dosage of pills. And will end up dozy, unable to think clearly, unsteady on his feet and yet still not able to sleep properly.

Third, there is evidence which suggests that the benzodiazepine drugs may make patients more susceptible to pain.

I firmly believe, therefore, that any pain patient who is suffering from insomnia and taking a sleeping tablet should try to wean him or herself off the sleeping tablets. Sleeping tablets never provide a long-term solution and rarely help. They usually cause far more problems than they solve. Since drugs of this type are potentially addictive it is essential that patients planning on stopping their tablets cut down slowly. My book *Life Without Tranquillisers* (published in paperback by Corgi) contains advice on how to give up tranquillizers.

2. Carefully assess your daily sleeping habits. Patients who complain that they cannot get to sleep at night will sometimes confess that they take a two-hour nap in the afternoon. Other patients go to bed at nine o'clock in the evening and then express surprise when they wake up at five or six o'clock the following morning.

The amount of sleep we need varies from individual to

individual and from circumstances to circumstances. But very few of us need more than eight hours' sleep in any one twenty-four-hour period. And our need for sleep tends to diminish as we get older. An average sixty-year-old, for example, will probably need no more than six or seven hours' sleep a night.

If, like most people, you prefer to get your sleep at night, try to avoid sleeping at any other time of day, and try to avoid going to bed too early in the evening.

3. Try to ensure that you don't get woken up unnecessarily. There is nothing more annoying than having to struggle to get to sleep and then waking up an hour later because you need to empty your bladder or because you're hot.

Avoid alcohol, tea, coffee and other drinks during the evening (alcohol, tea and coffee are all stimulants and are likely to keep you awake). Empty your bladder before you go to bed.

If you smoke then don't smoke for at least an hour or two before you go to bed. And don't smoke in bed. Nicotine can have a stimulating effect which will help to keep you awake.

Make sure that you don't get woken up by feeling too hot, too cold or uncomfortable in any other way. If your bedroom is noisy it may be worth investing in some soundproofing (book shelves – with books – are excellent for this purpose), or double glazing on your bedroom windows, or some simple ear plugs.

And make sure that your bed is comfortable too. Many people struggle on all their lives on an uncomfortable bed. Visit one or two large department stores and try out as many beds as possible before you buy one. If you and your partner need beds of different springiness then you should be able to adapt one side of the bed by pushing a wooden board between the mattress and the bed springs, or by using twin mattresses of different types.

4. Help yourself get to sleep by following this simple but specially prepared regimen.
a. Switch on your electric blanket or put a hot water bottle in your bed.

b. An hour before you go to bed take twenty minutes' brisk exercise. Take a walk outside. Use an indoor exercise machine. Climb up and down your stairs. Do press-ups and leg-raising exercises. Try to raise a sweat. While exercising, think through any of your day's problems.

c. Take a notebook and pencil and write down all your problems and worries. Keep your notebook by your side from now on. Every time a new problem or thought pops into your head, get rid of it by writing it down for consideration in the morning.

d. If you feel hungry have two dry biscuits and half a glass or mugful of a warm, milk-based drink.

e. Spend ten or fifteen minutes relaxing in a warm bath. Allow your mind to float quite freely as you bathe. If any fresh thoughts or ideas pop into your head write them down in your notebook.

f. Go to bed with a relaxing and distracting book. This is designed to eradicate the day's troubles, fears and anxieties from your head. Make sure that before you get into bed you take any pain-killing tablets that have been prescribed for you. If you have used an electric blanket make sure that it is switched off and the plug is pulled out of the mains.

g. Finally, you can try losing yourself in a daydream. (See the section beginning on page 85.)

Keep as Busy as You Can

Our natural reaction to pain is to rest. Under some circumstances this is appropriate, sensible and possibly the only choice. If you have a severe pain brought on by a recent injury, or you have a heart pain, then rest is essential.

But unless your pain is severe, acute, unexplained and recent in onset you may well be doing yourself more harm than good by resting. Physical inactivity can result in the weakening of muscles, the deterioration of many of the body's essential organs and body tissues, and the development of pressure sores. Mental inactivity can make pain worse simply by reducing the amount of sensory input going into the brain. The inevitable consequence of this is that the patient becomes increasingly aware of the pain sensations which are being transmitted.

I shall deal with the advantages of physical activity in the section dealing with exercise (on pages 135–9), but here I want to concentrate on the importance of keeping your brain as active as possible.

One of the earliest pieces of research to show the value of keeping your mind active was done by Frederick Kanfer and David Goldfoot of the University of Oregon Medical School a few years ago. They took a number of volunteer students and divided them into several groups. Members of the first group of students were told to sit still, do nothing and keep their hands in ice water for as long as possible. Members of the second group were told to put their hands into ice water, but also told that they could watch a specially situated clock and use the clock to help them set themselves goals and objectives. Members of the third group of volunteers were given access to a slide projector and a series of slides. They were allowed to operate the projector with their free hand and look at as many slides as they liked.

The results of this experiment showed that when people in pain keep their minds busy they increase their pain tolerance level. The volunteers in the first group, the ones who were resting and not thinking about anything in particular, managed to keep their hands in the ice water for an average of 174 seconds. The volunteers in the second group, the ones who were watching the clock, managed to last out for 196 seconds. But the volunteers who were allowed to watch the slides managed to keep their hands in the ice water for 271 seconds.

It seems to me that the only sensible conclusion that can be drawn from this experiment (and from other similar experiments which have been performed) is that the chronic pain sufferer should do everything in his or her power to keep busy, occupied and 'distracted'.

One of the examples I can think of to illustrate the practical value of keeping busy concerns Dr John Bonica, probably the world's leading pain specialist. (I have described Dr Bonica's contribution more fully on page 61.) Dr Bonica suffers from very bad arthritis, his left leg is one and a half inches shorter than his right leg, and he has had numerous operations to correct arthritic deformities. He is in more or less constant pain and cannot stand without pain. And yet Dr Bonica still writes and lectures regularly, and still scuba-dives. His one concession to his infirmity is that he no longer water-skis every day. Dr Bonica confirms that by staying active he helps to keep his pain under control.

Pain Control Programme prescription

1. Many hospitals run occupational therapy departments these days, but unfortunately occupational therapists aren't always able to provide all their patients with demanding or inspiring activities. There is, in some areas at least, still too much emphasis on basket weaving, embroidery and pottery.

You'll benefit far more if you can get yourself back to work and start fitting into a regular, albeit demanding, routine.

Once you've been off work for two years or more, getting back into the routine can be difficult so, despite your pain, try to get back into the swing of things as soon as you possibly can. Work is likely to provide you with physical activity, mental stimulation and something to inspire your enthusiasm as well as your interest. The financial rewards will also help to enable you to satisfy your other needs and ambitions.

A research paper read at the International Association for the Study of Pain's Second World Congress on Pain in Montreal, Canada, in the summer of 1978, and written by Toshihiko Maruta, David Swanson and Wendell Swenson suggested that patients who had lost more than one and a half years from work through their pain were often particularly difficult to help.

2. If you need more intellectual stimulation in your life, or you feel the need for new friends, then start taking evening classes or day classes at a local college. Don't just pick a subject that sounds useful. Try to find something that excites you and that you will enjoy. If it's useful as well, consider that a bonus.

3. If you find yourself in a situation where you need to keep your mind busy in order to escape from pain but where it is not possible to read a book, watch a television programme or get on with some work (for example, when you are sitting in a dentist's chair) then escape by creating fantasy daydreams for yourself. Think of a situation that you would enjoy, of people you would like to be with, and of places you would like to visit. Then add as much exotic (or erotic) background to the fantasy as you like. Create an invigorating, exciting fantasy.

Fantasize about success, about what you would do if you won half a million pounds on the football pools, about what it would be like to have a motor yacht moored at Monaco, about what it would be like to own a stately home, about what it would be like to trek across the Himalayas.

If you have difficulty in creating suitable fantasies for yourself, collect a pile of brochures from a travel agent or buy one or two absurd magazines from your newsagents. A journal full of pictures of elegant country houses, expensive boats or strange lands should provide a useful starting point.

4. When you need to distract yourself from your pain, create mental games to keep your mind occupied. Try doing mental arithmetic. Try counting the number of cracks in the ceiling at the dentist's surgery. Try counting the number of patterns on the wallpaper in your bedroom. It doesn't really matter what you do as long as you keep your mind busy.

Be Prepared to Assert Yourself

In 1962 two researchers called Lazarus and Abramovitz stated that according to their studies patients suffering from physical or mental problems produced by anxiety could help themselves by becoming more self-assertive or by building up their sense of personal pride.

A year or two later in another experiment Gretchen Timmermans of the Pain Unit at the Veterans Administration Hospital in San Diego, California, and Richard Sternback of the Department of Psychiatry at the University of California studied 119 patients suffering from persistent, long-lasting pain and concluded that many patients who suffer from persistent pain admit that they find it difficult to talk about their feelings and that they find their anger being bottled up inside themselves. Other researchers then showed that anxiety makes pain worse too. It was only a matter of time before researchers put these separate themes together and looked for evidence showing that assertiveness can be used to help inhibit the sort of anxiety responses likely to result in the development or exacerbation of pain.

It was in an experiment conducted by Thomas Westcott of Western Carolina University and John Horan of Pennsylvania State University that it was first shown that when patients in pain are made to feel angry and encouraged to assert themselves then they can improve their ability to cope with their pain. The experiment they conducted in order to obtain their evidence involved the now almost traditional ice water test.

In the first part of the experiment a group of volunteers were told to put their dominant hands into nine inches of ice water and to hold their hands there for as long as possible.

In the second part of the experiment Horan and Westcott did what they could to make their volunteers feel angry and assertive. While their hands were in the ice water the volunteers were allowed to listen to a very short recorded drama designed to make them feel angry and self-righteous.

It worked. And the results were very impressive – particularly for the women who took part in the tests. When instructed to keep their hands in icy water for as long as they could manage the women could keep their hands submerged only for a modest 70 seconds. But when they were allowed to listen to the recorded drama the women managed a remarkable 268 seconds.

Since then other research workers have confirmed not only that patients are more susceptible to pain when their self-esteem is low and when they are unable to express their anger, but that patients who build up their self-confidence and who learn to assert themselves can increase their tolerance of pain and their ability to withstand pain.

There have been a number of clinical reports from doctors who have indeed shown that it is the patients who do not assert themselves who are the patients who are most likely to suffer from intractable and difficult pain and the ones who are first to die. The patients who are considered to be 'model' patients and who are widely liked by all the doctors and nurses looking after them are the ones who don't survive.

The patients who survive and suffer least pain are the patients who are aggressive, who refuse to be dominated, who want to be put into a good position near to the window and won't readily accept administrative nonsense just because everyone else accepts it, who demand information and make notes of what they are told, who want to know the reason behind every test and procedure and who, in short, stick up for themselves as individuals. Doctors and nurses understandably like their patients to be unassertive – it makes the hospital easier to run if all the patients keep still and don't ask too many questions. But patients suffer less pain if they stick up for themselves. The patients who fight, who demand to be allowed out of bed, who demand to be allowed home, may not be the most popular patients among the hospital staff but they tend to be the patients who survive and who need the smallest quantities of pain killers.

Clearly, therefore, if you feel that you have difficulty in expressing your anger, if you suspect that you don't assert yourself enough or if you believe that you lack self-confidence, you would undoubtedly be able to improve your ability both to control your pain and to cope with it by learning how to assert yourself a little more forcibly and by learning to express your anger when it is building up inside you.

Pain Control Programme prescription

The first thing to remember if you are going to assert yourself is that you don't have to become rude or unpleasant. You simply have to become more aware of your own needs and wishes, and more prepared to stand your ground when you are being put under pressure by someone else.

1. Start by learning how to stop other people manipulating you. Learn how to say 'No' when people are pushing you into doing things that you really don't want to do. Try to get into the habit of asserting yourself and seeing yourself as an assertive and independent individual.

Imagine, for example, that you are at a dinner party and your hostess wants you to have another helping when you really couldn't eat another thing. If you are the non-assertive, compliant sort of individual then you'll probably end up eating food you really don't want or need simply in order to avoid upsetting your hostess.

Try to imagine that you're sitting at the dinner table and that the most forceful hostess you know is pressing you to take another helping. And that you're full and really don't want anything else to eat. Imagine that you can see yourself saying 'No' in a forceful and very polite and flattering way. Instead of offering a bald 'No, thank you' hear yourself saying something like 'No, thank you. It was absolutely delicious but I really couldn't eat another thing.'

If you think about it carefully then you'll realize that if

your hostess still tries to force you to accept more food then she is being unreasonable and rude. Imagine that you are an outsider looking in at the dinner party. Could you possibly fault your own behaviour? Of course you couldn't. You have no need to feel guilty or ashamed because you've had enough to eat.

And if your hostess ignores your request and simply puts food on to your plate then just see yourself putting down your knife and fork on the side of your plate and leaving the food uneaten. The chances are that your hostess will be so busy trying to push food on to some other unfortunate victim that she won't even notice what you've done anyway.

The more you run this scene through your mind the more you will be able to assert yourself next time a similar situation arises. Every time you imagine yourself being successfully self-assertive then you will build up your courage, self-confidence and ability to assert yourself. The self-confidence that you have built up in this simple way will help you deal with other far more complex and far more difficult situations.

2. You can also help yourself considerably by learning to build up your confidence in your own abilities and skills. Many of the people who suffer serious pain because of their inability to assert themselves have a very low opinion of their own skills and qualities.

The fact is, however, that if you lack confidence then the chances are that although you know very well what your weaknesses are you don't know what your strengths are. You are probably rather timid and shy (even though other people may not realize that), and doubtless you have little faith in your own abilities.

To counteract those fears, sit down with a piece of paper and a pencil and write down all the good things you can think of to say about yourself. Imagine that you are preparing an advertising campaign for yourself. Throw modesty out of the window and try to promote all your virtues and good points. Imagine that you're trying to sell yourself to the world.

You'll probably be amazed to see just how many virtues you've got. Individuals who are shy and lacking in self-confidence tend to be unusually honest, generous, thoughtful and hard-working. You're probably punctual, careful, moral, kind, ambitious and unusually creative.

3. When you are next feeling low in self-confidence make a list of all your assets. I don't mean a crude list of the money you have and the things you own, but a list of all the intangibles in your life: your partner, your children, your integrity, your friends, your interests, your knowledge, your accomplishments and your memories – particularly your memories. Those are the real valuables in your life.

4. Learn to deal with your anger in as positive and as practical a way as possible. Don't just let it build up inside you. You have to learn to accept the fact that you, like everyone else, will get angry from time to time. Anger is a perfectly natural and reasonably healthy response to stressful circumstances. Anger becomes a destructive and dangerous problem only when it is allowed to build up inside you. It is no sin to acknowledge the existence of your anger and to let it out occasionally.

If you feel yourself getting angry ask yourself whether or not the matter is worth getting angry about and whether or not your anger is justified. If your answer to both these questions is 'Yes' then don't suppress your anger or try to hide it. Let it out. And if you feel your anger building up inside you and you feel tempted to get rid of your anger in some direct, physical way, then follow your natural instincts just as much as possible.

I'm not, of course, suggesting that you race round and hit anyone who has annoyed you. That wouldn't be very practical. But you can get rid of your excess anger by hitting a squash or tennis ball, by kicking a football, by smashing your fist into a punch bag, by beating a carpet, by digging the garden, by breaking twigs for the fire or even by taking a pile of old plates into the garage and smashing them one by one.

5. Many people whose pain is made worse by their feelings

of inadequacy habitually criticize themselves and 'put themselves down'. Try to decide whether you ever do this.

Do you, for example, say things like 'I'm no good at that', or 'I'm just a very ordinary person?' Do you constantly find yourself apologizing for your behaviour or your weaknesses?

If you do then you should try to break the habit permanently. Every time you find yourself saying or thinking something negative and self-deprecatory say '*Stop!*' to yourself. Then say or think something positive and encouraging. Remind yourself of your skills and strengths, your good qualities and your virtues.

Learning How to Rest

As I have explained elsewhere in this book (see page 101) it is a mistake to rest too much. If you suffer regularly from pain you must stay as active as you possibly can. If you rest too much your body and your mind will both stagnate. Your muscles and other tissues will atrophy and the sharp cutting edges of your mind will become dull and blunt.

But there are times when rest is important, and it is important that any pain sufferer knows when to rest and how to rest.

Pain Control Programme prescription

1. You must know *when* your body really needs rest, and when too much activity will make your pain worse rather than better.

The most important thing to remember is that whenever you have an acute or sudden attack of pain you should try to rest. You should certainly avoid doing anything which makes your pain worse or which exacerbates any other aspect of your condition. This does not mean that you should never move any part of your body that is in pain. It is, for example, often vital to keep moving joints that are sore and painful. If you do not move them then they will deteriorate even more. You should, however, be able to differentiate between genuine and threatening pain and modest and bearable discomfort.

In addition you should also be prepared to rest when you feel tired or exhausted or worn out. Some people who suffer from pain are so determined to keep mobile and active that they force themselves to keep moving all the time. Some people who suffer from persistent pain or recurrent pain constantly push themselves to do more and more.

It is important to keep active and busy, but if you try to force your body to do too much then you will exhaust yourself and increase your susceptibility to pain. It is important that you know your limits and that you are prepared to take a rest when you feel that your body needs a break.

2. You must also know *how* to rest so that your body benefits fully.

When you have an acute attack of pain you should simply do your best to manoeuvre yourself into as comfortable a position as possible.

Do not, however, be tempted to put pillows under sore joints or hold limbs in fixed positions. If you do then there is a real risk that your joint will become fixed and immobile in a difficult and impractical position. Remember that painful joints can become stiff very quickly.

When you have a longer-term need for rest, you should plan your rest with care and caution. One of the best and more effective ways of dealing with exhaustion is to change your way of life temporarily and take a few days away from all your problems. You may find that if you elect to take a few days in the country or at the seaside you will be able to leave many of your problems and pains behind you.

Sadly, many people who are trying to rest make the mistake of spending their valuable and often stolen days of respite struggling to accumulate a series of exotic experiences and photographs with which they can impress their neighbours. This is a dreadful mistake.

If you need a rest and you decide to go off camping for a few days then you'll probably merely exchange one set of problems for another set of problems. There really isn't very much point in trying to escape from the problems of a stress-ridden city life if you merely end up spending all your time sheltering from the rain and trying to cook a three-course meal on a one-ring Primus stove.

If you're planning a break because you need a rest then make sure that you do something that will allow you to unwind. Go to a hotel or boarding house where you can behave as casually as you like. Don't give yourself any targets or things to see. Take a few books with you if you like, but ensure that you will not be under any pressure while you are away.

If you think that your pain will benefit from a break, remember that you need to rest both your body and your mind.

How Massage Can Help You

Massage has been popular for thousands of years and is of more value than most of us imagine. In recent years postcard-sized advertisements in seedy shop windows have given massage a rather bad name. However, massage can help ease tension, soothe tight muscles and relieve pain extremely effectively. Massage helps in a number of quite specific ways.

First, it helps to clear away the knots that accumulate in your muscles when you are anxious or nervous. Normally when you feel tense your muscles tighten as part of your natural response to stress and fear. Your body responds in this way because it assumes that a physical response will help you deal with your stress – indeed, if you are facing a genuine physical threat then it will help if your muscles are ready for action: you'll be better able to run, jump, climb or fight.

Unfortunately, of course, most of our problems these days can't be dealt with by a purely physical response. And so the physical response is inappropriate. Even more important is the fact that as your problems and worries and tensions persist, so does your muscle tension. And as the tension persists, so the muscles stay contracted and waste products such as lactic acid accumulate. These accumulated wastes worsen things by making your muscles stiff and painful and preventing them from relaxing.

By massaging these areas (and most commonly muscle tension seems to affect the muscles in the neck, shoulders and back) it is possible to clear away the accumulated wastes, and to relieve muscle stiffness. A good massage can clear knots out of muscles just as surely as it is possible to clear the wrinkles from a bed sheet by gentle stroking.

Second, the personal contact that is an inevitable part of a massage helps too. In our society we touch one another comparatively little; social rules and requirements make it unacceptable for us to touch strangers or even to touch loved ones in public. And yet there is a good deal of evidence to show that we need to be touched and to touch one another. Children who are not cuddled or touched by their parents as they are growing up will develop all sorts of emotional problems – the same thing happens with young animals too. Gentle massage can help relieve pain and tension by providing sympathy and reassurance.

Third, there are some doctors and psychologists who believe that by relaxing muscles through massage a masseur doesn't just have an effect on the body but has a very positive soothing effect on the mind too. Wilhelm Reich, a psychologist who practised at the turn of the century, believed that some people hide their emotions in their muscles and that there is a strong link between the two. Just what the link consists of is a mystery, but it is certainly true that many people do feel mentally relaxed and comfortable after a massage.

Finally, and perhaps most important of all, there is evidence that massage has two very specific and positive pain-relieving effects. It helps to stimulate the production of endorphins, the body's internally produced pain-relieving hormones. And by stimulating the production of sensory impulses which will be carried along the body's larger nerve fibres it blocks the transmission of pain messages by closing the gate at the spinal cord.

An additional advantage is that when you are able to move your muscles and joints more freely after massage your brain will start sending instructions down your spinal cord to your muscles; those descending impulses also play a part in keeping the spinal cord gateway closed to pain impulses.

Pain Control Programme prescription

1. There are many different types of massage, and it is worth knowing a little about some of the most popular technical

terms that are used. I have, therefore, compiled a glossary of some of the best-known types of massage.

EFFLEURAGE
Soothing massage movements are usually described as effleurage. The flat of the hand is used to stroke the muscles. The aim is to improve the circulation and prepare the muscles for a more aggressive, vigorous massage.

FRICTION MASSAGE
Friction massage involves rubbing the skin with the fingers.

PETRISSAGE
This involves pinching, kneading and rolling the skin. In this way larger muscles are relaxed and the general skin condition is said to be improved.

TAPOTEMENT
This form of massage involves beating, whipping, slapping and tapping the skin in order to stimulate and tighten it.

VIBRATION MASSAGE
Vibration massage involves a delicate tapping and circling of the skin with the fingertips to stimulate the circulation. Electric vibrators are also sometimes used (see also pages 127–8); but note that with these there is a risk that the subcutaneous tissues may be damaged if the massage is not done carefully. This type of massage is often done to relieve tension.

SWEDISH MASSAGE
The phrase 'Swedish massage' always seems to attract giggles and knowing looks. In fact 'Swedish massage' is a phrase used to describe the sort of service usually offered in topless massage parlours. The name is presumably derived from the fact that the Swedes are supposed to enjoy pretty free love lives.

2. It is possible to obtain a good massage in most towns or cities these days. Most health farms or large hotels can give you the name and telephone number of a reliable local

masseur (or masseuse). Health clubs, swimming baths and gyms are another possibility. Or you could try telephoning numbers from the Yellow Pages, or from advertisements in your local newspaper. But do make it clear that you want a massage to relieve your pain (a relief massage is something quite different).

3. Do remember that there is a tremendous difference between massage and manipulation. The former simply involves the rubbing, kneading and rolling of the skin and muscles. The latter involves stretching and twisting joints. You should not allow anyone other than a qualified doctor or osteopath to manipulate your bones and joints. (There are many untested theories about just how manipulation works. Some osteopaths claim to be able to replace bones in the correct position, some say that they are releasing trapped air pockets in joints, while a third claim is that manipulation breaks up scar tissue. I have no idea whether any of these theories are correct or not but there is no doubt that under some circumstances manipulation can help a considerable amount.)

4. Massage should never be painful, although when relieving stiffness it may occasionally prove slightly uncomfortable. If you're having a massage and it hurts then tell the masseur to stop and be more gentle.

5. Although it can be extremely pleasant to have a massage from a skilled professional you don't have to visit a professional in order to benefit from a massage: you can simply persuade a friend or relative to give you one. For a home massage follow these simple instructions.

First, you must make sure that you both feel completely comfortable. Any clothes that either of you wear should be loose and light and the room temperature should be pleasantly warm. If the temperature is too low your muscles will contract and become stiff and difficult to massage. The room should not be too light, so simply use a small bedside lamp or table lamp for illumination. You may both find gentle background music helpful and relaxing.

Second, although a massage couch is obviously ideal, very few homes have anything comparable to the equipment likely to be available in a professional's studio. A bed or springy sofa will be useless since there will be far too much bounce in either. The most satisfactory solution is for the person who is to have the massage to lie down flat on the floor. A foam mat or a couple of rugs spread out on the carpet should be enough to make things acceptably comfortable. If you're going to use oil or powder during the massage then it is a good idea to spread an old sheet over the carpet to catch any mess.

Third, if you're going to have the front of your body massaged put one small cushion under your head and another under your knees. If you're going to have your back massaged you won't need any cushions.

Fourth, remember that oil lubricates the skin and makes it much easier to give a massage. (If you don't like oil use talcum powder, which works almost as well.) You can buy very light, easily absorbed massage oils. Some experts believe that if special aromatic oils are massaged into the skin they will produce a healing effect on the body. I don't think that you need bother about any of these claims. I am perfectly happy to accept that an aromatic massage may be pleasant, but I know of no convincing evidence to show that it is especially therapeutic or particularly beneficial.

Fifth, don't be put off if neither of you knows much about massage. The person giving the massage should simply follow his or her intuition. A lot of nonsense is talked by people who want to turn massage into a full-blown profession. The fact is that you can benefit a tremendous amount by simply learning the necessary techniques as you go along. Start with a general massage involving all areas of the body and concentrate your massage attempts on those specific parts of the body which are particularly sore or tense. It is worth remembering that pounding, slapping or kneading a sore area of the body will often prove to be extremely beneficial. Do, however, remember to be cautious when moving joints and to avoid the spine completely.

6. If you think you'd benefit from a massage but you haven't

got a close friend or relative willing or able to give you a massage then don't despair: you can always give yourself one. You won't be able to reach all parts of your back, of course, but you will be able to reach many of the parts of your body which are most likely to benefit from massage. After all most of us automatically stretch our aching backs and rub those parts of our bodies that ache; when we do this we are instinctively helping ourselves through a simple form of massage therapy.

7. Here are some tips worth remembering.

First, if you have a headache or a painful stiff neck, you can help yourself an enormous amount by kneading your shoulders and the back of your neck with your fingers. You can also help yourself get rid of a headache by massaging the area just between your eyes, the areas to the side of your eyes and the areas just in front of your ears.

Second, next time you're washing your hair give your scalp a really thorough massage. You'll find it marvellously relaxing and soothing.

Third, you can massage your feet quite easily and your hands very easily. The alternative medical speciality of reflexology depends upon the theory that by massaging different parts of the hands and feet it is possible to influence organs and tissues deep inside your body. I'm not sure how much truth there is in this theory, but it certainly is true that a good hand or foot massage will relieve all sorts of pains and discomforts. Simply work your way over your hands and feet, working your way inwards from the tips of your fingers and toes to the palm of your hand and the ball of your foot. Massaging your feet doesn't tickle if it's done firmly, by the way.

Fourth, get a cat. Stroking a cat is particularly relaxing and soothing because when you stroke the cat you are inevitably stroking your hand at the same time; that stimulates the production of nervous impulses which pass along the larger nerve fibres and block the passage of pain messages. Since cats are warm creatures, you benefit from the heat they produce too.

The TENS Machine

Using electricity to relieve pain is nothing new. Ancient Egyptians and Hippocrates are said to have used electricity and in AD 46 a Roman physician called Scribonius Largus is credited with having claimed to be able to cure headaches with the energy produced by an electric torpedo fish.

After that promising start the role of electricity in medicine was forgotten for the best part of two thousand years. Then in the middle part of the nineteenth century it once again became fashionable to talk about electricity as a pain-relieving aid. All sorts of wonderful gadgets were put on the market, and excessive claims were made by the manufacturers.

The real value of electricity as a pain reliever was really only discovered fairly recently, however, and came about only after the gate control theory, put forward by Melzack and Wall, became fairly widely accepted.

As I've already described in an earlier section of this book (see page 14) the gate control theory suggests that when the skin or tissues are damaged messages carrying information about the injury travel towards the brain along two quite separate sets of nerve fibres. The larger fibres carry messages about sensations other than pain, and the smaller nerve fibres carry pain messages. The messages travelling along the large fibres tend to arrive at the spinal cord before the messages travelling along the smaller fibres and, if there are enough non-painful sensations travelling, the pain messages won't be able to get through.

Once Melzack and Wall had produced this theory it was possible to explain all sorts of natural phenomena that had up until that time been rather a mystery to physiologists. So, for example, it became clear that when we rub a sore spot, what we are doing is increasing the number of non-painful messages travelling towards the spinal cord's nerve gateway. If you knock your elbow you'll automatically reach to rub the spot because subconsciously you know that by rubbing the area you'll be able to cut down the amount of pain that you feel.

Having realized just how rubbing a sore spot can relieve pain, the next step was for scientists to come up with a way of stimulating the passage of non-painful sensations quite automatically. They had the idea of using electricity to produce the necessary stimulus.

When the theory was first put into practice in the late 1960s doctors suggested that the electricity should be introduced into the body through electrodes surgically implanted into the spine. Although that did seem to work, the fact that it involved a surgical operation (though only a minor one) limited the usefulness and availability of the procedure.

The next development made the whole concept much more readily available. It was discovered that all nerves within an inch or two of the surface of the skin can be stimulated by electrodes which are simply stuck on to the skin.

And that was exactly what the next teams of researchers started doing. They started giving patients pocket-sized battery-operated stimulators which sent out a continuous series of electrical pulses and which could transmit those pulses into the large nerves of the body via silicon electrodes stuck on to the skin with a special conducting paste. And it worked.

Moreover, it was found that Transcutaneous Electrical Nerve Stimulation (it quickly became known as TENS for obvious reasons) didn't just stimulate the passage of sensory impulses designed to inhibit the passage of pain impulses; it also stimulated the body to start producing its own pain-relieving hormones, the endorphins.

Obviously the next step was to start conducting experiments to see how effective TENS was. During the last decade an impressive number of projects have been undertaken and have shown without doubt that TENS is extremely effective in relieving pain.

In a study conducted with patients suffering from rheumatoid arthritis it was found that the TENS equipment produced pain relief in up to 95 per cent of patients. In other experiments it was found that TENS even managed to produce relief in patients who had received no relief from any other pain-relieving techniques. Dr John Bonica has said that TENS provides relief for 65 to 80 per cent of all pain patients in the short term, and long-term relief for between 30 and 50 per cent of patients. According to Professor John Thompson, Professor of Pharmacology at the University of Newcastle-upon-Tyne, who is consultant clinical pharmacologist for the Newcastle Health Authority and consultant in charge at the pain relief clinic at the Royal Victoria Infirmary in Newcastle, short-term improvement after using TENS may be between 80 and 90 per cent with a very respectable 35 per cent of patients still benefiting from pain relief after two years' use. It has been shown that the TENS machine is good for relieving low back pain, phantom limb pain, arthritis of all kinds, cancer pain and the pain that sometimes develops after herpes. A large study done in Sweden has shown that TENS is the only pain killer required by 70 per cent of women in labour. It works well for patients recovering from surgery too. There are extremely few side effects or problems caused by TENS and the cost of running the machines is low.

With this sort of success available from a small portable machine that can be bought quite cheaply and used at home without very much training, you'd imagine that doctors all around the world would be recommending TENS to their patients.

They aren't. And the drug companies are, perhaps not surprisingly, not very keen on TENS. It could virtually destroy their multi-million pound sales of pain killers every year.

If you suspect that I'm being too cynical, consider this short story. In 1970 two men, Norman Hagfors and Stanley McDonald, working in the basement of Mr Hagfors's home in Minneapolis, invented an early electronic pain killer. The two men had previously worked with a company which manufactured pacemakers, and they were familiar with the medical practice of implanting electrodes into patients' spines in order to block the transmission of pain signals to the brain.

But they thought that they could make a machine that would have the same effect without needing surgery – in effect an early TENS machine.

With the aid of electrical components bought at a local hardware shop Hagfors and McDonald built a small device which did exactly what they'd hoped: it blocked pain simply through electrodes stuck on the skin. Within three years the company the two men had formed, Stimulation Technology Inc., was selling almost a million dollars' worth of the devices every year.

Then in 1974 one of the world's big pharmaceutical manufacturers bought out the company for $1.3 million, promising the two inventors a share of the future profits. But, according to Hagfors and McDonald, the drug company did little or nothing to promote the product to pain sufferers, even though clinical trials had been successful.

Despite the lack of enthusiasm from doctors and the undoubted opposition from various parts of the drug industry, TENS machines *are* available. At the last count there were something like forty different companies making TENS machines and selling them, often for no more than the cost of a portable radio, to hundreds of thousands of pain sufferers.

Pain Control Programme prescription

If you want to try a TENS device then you'll probably have to buy one for, although there are some doctors and clinics who have these machines available for their patients to try out on loan, there is virtually no chance of your being able to obtain one on permanent loan. For some strange reason doctors are allowed to prescribe millions of pounds' worth of unnecessary pain killers (and contribute to the healthy profits of the international drug industry) but they are not allowed to prescribe TENS machines for their patients to use.

If you want to buy yourself a TENS machine then I suggest that you start by asking your doctor if he has one he can lend you or if he knows whether your local hospital has any available for patients to try. You may be lucky. If there are no TENS machines available in your area then you'll have to buy one. All I can suggest you do is look in your local Yellow Pages for your nearest medical equipment supplier. Then ask him to let you see a copy of his catalogue. It's also worth asking whether he has any machines available on sale or return. Some manufacturers will refund part of the purchase price if customers do not obtain any pain relief.

Once you have your machine, you'll probably have to experiment with it a little before you obtain any useful effect. First read the manufacturer's instructions and follow them very carefully.

There are two variables with every TENS device: the strength of the electrical pulse being produced by the machine and the position where the electrodes are applied.

Getting the level of stimulation right is fairly straight-forward. All you have to do is increase the stimulation until it produces pain and then turn it down until it is comfortable. When you feel a pleasant and acceptable tingling, the machine is set.

Finding the right place for the electrodes is more difficult. Some machines have two electrodes, others have four simply to give you double the chance to stimulate the appropriate nerves. Most experts recommend that you begin by placing the electrodes on the points of greatest tenderness. If stimulating them for thirty minutes or so doesn't help relieve your pain then you should simply move the electrodes over the painful area until you find a spot where they do work. Or you can try pressing your skin with your fingers until you find tender spots, and then stick your electrodes over those points.

The TENS device suppresses your pain not only at the time but also, it seems, long after the machine has been switched off. Many patients find that they can free themselves of pain more or less completely by using their device as little as two or three times a week. Others find that they need to keep their device in place permanently and use it virtually all the time.

Apart from the fact that TENS shouldn't be used by pregnant women (because it's always wise to be cautious if you're pregnant) or by people who have a heart pacemaker, and that you shouldn't try to use one if you're driving, and that you shouldn't use it around your eyes, there aren't really any dangers or problems with it. The commonest side effect seems to be a slight skin rash caused by the jelly used to stick the electrodes to the skin.

Finally, two things worth remembering about TENS. First, it seems to work best with persistent and fairly stable pains: headaches, stiff necks, backaches, joint pains and period pains, for example, rather than pains that are sudden, acute or shooting. And second, even though TENS doesn't always cut out pain completely it very often relieves it enough to enable a disabled or bedbound patient to become an active member of the community again. If a TENS device can make the difference between lying in bed and living a fairly normal life then the investment has to be worthwhile.

Let's hope that the politicians see sense before too long and make TENS devices freely available on prescription. Health costs would plummet if they did, for the savings on pain-killing tablets would be phenomenal. TENS devices are safe, effective and economical, but their ultimate advantage is that they work not by attacking the body but by stimulating the body's own pain-suppressing mechanisms.

The Rocking Chair

According to Dr Barry Wyke, director of the Royal College of Surgeons Neurological Unit, one of the most effective ways of managing chronic low back pain in elderly patients is to tell them to sit in a rocking chair and 'rock around the clock'.

According to a report in the journal *Pain Topics*, Dr Wyke told a back pain research symposium that using a rocking chair stimulates the production of nerve impulses which provide effective and continuous pain relief. Dr Wyke even went so far as to claim that the increase in back pain that has caused so much misery this century may be partly due to the disappearance of the rocking chair.

I'm not sure that I'd go quite that far, but I certainly think that there is plenty of evidence to show that a rocking chair can help relieve pains of many different kinds. It is soothing, restful and relaxing. Those who think of the rocking chair as a completely old-fashioned piece of furniture might be interested to know that John Kennedy, who suffered from chronic backache, spent many hours sitting in the soothing comfort of a rocking chair when working in the White House.

Pain Control Programme prescription

Buy a comfortable rocking chair and use it as often as you can. Since pain tends to get worse during the evening, it's a good idea to sit in your rocking chair if you are watching television or relaxing.

The Vibrator

Stroking and rubbing a sore area helps to control pain by stimulating the production of sensory nerve impulses which travel quickly along the larger nerve fibres, get to the gate in the spinal cord first and block the passageway of pain impulses. The TENS device works in exactly the same way.

If you can't afford a TENS device, or you don't want to buy one, then you may be able to obtain a very similar effect by using a vibrator – exactly the same sort of hand-held vibrator as is sold in sex shops for other purposes.

According to Dr David Ottoson, from the Karolinska Institute in Stockholm, Sweden, when an ordinary sex shop vibrator was used by seventeen patients suffering from trigeminal neuralgia (a severe type of facial pain) and held on the painful part of their faces for thirty minutes, fourteen of them reported that their pain was reduced significantly both during stimulation and for some time afterwards. Eight out of the seventeen patients reported that they obtained relief for four to six hours afterwards. These patients had all had their pain for some time (in some cases a number of years) and all reported that the vibrator was more effective than anything else they had tried. Most important of all, a year after the initial experiment the patients were still getting benefit from their vibrators.

In another research project conducted at a Swedish dental clinic forty-seven out of fifty patients with tooth pain reported that they obtained relief by holding a vibrator on or near the painful part of their face for thirty minutes or so.

Pain Control Programme prescription

Buy yourself a small vibrator. You may be able to find a surgical supplies store which sells vibrators. Alternatively, you can buy one from a sex shop or by mail order.

Use the vibrator by holding it against the area of your pain for thirty minutes or so at a time. You may need to repeat this three times a day.

Heat Treatment

Heat has been used to help relieve pain for centuries, and just about every country in the world has a history of using spas, saunas, hot springs, baths and soaking tubs to help eradicate pain. Although heat can help just about any type of pain it seems to work best for the sort of pain produced by bruises, tears, strains and joint inflammation.

Just how it produces its useful effect is still something of a mystery, although scientists have put forward several theories. It has been suggested that heat generates nerve impulses which help close down the gate in the spinal cord and stop pain impulses getting through. Alternatively, it could be that since it is the responsibility of the blood to remove products such as prostaglandins and histamine (chemicals which are produced by the body and which are responsible for the sensation of pain) and, since heating the tissues increases the flow of the blood, heating the body may increase the rate at which pain disappears.

The truth is that both these theories are probably correct, although to a certain extent the question of just how heat relieves pain is rather academic since the important thing is that we know that heat *does* relieve pain.

Pain Control Programme prescription

There are numerous ways of applying heat to your body if you want to relieve pain. The best way is probably by having a warm bath. Millions of gardeners and sportsmen will confirm that nothing soothes sore and inflamed muscles quite as much as lying down in a bathful of warm water. As an alternative to an ordinary hot bath you could try visiting your nearest spa, sauna, steam room or well-heated swimming pool.

If you want to apply heat to specific areas of your body then you can try using heated towels, an electrically-heated pad, a sun lamp or an old-fashioned hot-water bottle. If you use a hot-water bottle, make sure that the rubber is not perished, that the stopper fits well and that the bottle is wrapped in a towel so that it does not burn your skin.

Ice Treatment

Few of us think of ice as being a useful remedy for pain. Indeed, many times in this book I have described experiments in which ice has been used to *cause* pain under experimental conditions. Nevertheless, the fact is that cold is often even more effective than heat at relieving pain.

So, for example, Dr Gerald Aronoff, Director of Boston Pain Clinic at Massachusetts Rehabilitation Hospital, has claimed that after being massaged with ice many patients get up to four hours of pain relief. In a study Dr Aronoff conducted with fifty patients at his Boston clinic he found that 78 per cent of patients with lower back pain and headaches reported obtaining significant pain relief while another 8 per cent got some relief by using ice. In another study involving patients with dental pain, ice massage produced relief in over half of the patients.

Several theories have been put forward to try and explain how ice works as a pain reliever. One theory is that it produces local constrictions of blood vessels and makes the area feel numb. Another theory is that ice works in much the same way as TENS, by producing endorphins and interfering with the passage of pain impulses.

Pain Control Programme prescription

1. Ice is particularly good for bruises, headaches, painful limbs, joint problems, backache and muscle pain.

2. To avoid being cut by pieces of ice which are sharp-edged, put ice cubes into a rubber ice bag or hot-water bottle; or put

a lollipop stick into a paper cup of water and freeze it; or pour water into a small bowl, freeze it and then get rid of the hard edges by running hot water over the ice block. As a final alternative you can simply wrap ice cubes in a thin cloth such as a tea towel.

3. Obtain ice relief by rubbing ice on the skin all over the painful area in circular or backwards-and-forwards movements. Press fairly firmly. When you rub ice on your skin you should first feel the cold, then feel a burning, then a stiffness and finally a numbing. You should not hold ice in contact with your skin for more than five minutes at a time. Remember that ice – like heat – can burn. You should keep the ice moving so that it does not remain in contact with one part of your skin for more that a few seconds. As soon as your skin feels numb, remove the ice and start to move the area immediately. You should notice that the area is more easily moved than before.

Counter-irritation

Many traditional methods of providing pain relief depend on the theory that if you irritate the skin in some way then you will not notice your original pain. In addition, it is believed that if you irritate the skin the flow of blood through the local tissues will be increased, with the result that the accumulating pain-producing hormones will be removed more speedily.

Some of the old-fashioned methods of irritating the skin to obtain this effect are rather drastic. At various times in history people have put hot metal rods on to their skin, cut their skin with sharp knives, applied a mustard plaster to the painful area and tried deliberately bruising their skin by using a technique known as 'cupping'.

I don't think cupping has much of a place in late twentieth-century medicine but it is worth a brief mention. You simply pour hot water into an ordinary cup so that the cup itself becomes heated, then you empty the water out of the cup and place the open mouth of the cup directly onto your skin. As the cup cools the air inside contracts and sucks your skin into the cup, damaging it slightly in the process. The area then becomes slightly painful. The theory is that because you've become aware of your new pain you'll forget your original pain.

Today the most common way to conquer pain by counter-irritation is to rub a liniment or rubefacient onto your skin. There are all sorts of products available in this general category, and they work by making an area of skin feel hot and rather irritated. Presumably, the passage of sensory impulses along the large nerve fibres combines with the effect of the heat that has been produced to suppress the sensation of pain.

Pain Control Programme prescription

1. There are numerous liniments readily available. Oil of wintergreen is one of the best known. To use one of these liniments you simply rub a small amount on to the skin over your aching joint or muscles. The area will soon feel warm, and may go red as the blood flow increases. If you have sensitive or eczematous skin then you should be particularly careful when using a liniment.

If you intend to try a liniment or rubefacient, be careful not to take aspirin at or around the same time. A liniment works by producing redness and heat in the skin. But aspirin tablets work by opposing those very same effects and counteracting the type of inflammation produced by a liniment. In a report published in the *British Medical Journal* in 1985 a group of haematologists working in Glasgow reported that patients who take aspirin and use a liniment obtain absolutely no useful effect; the two products simply cancel one another out.

The Importance of Exercise

If you are in pain there is a tremendous temptation to avoid exercise at all costs. Understandable though this may be, it can be a mistake.

Naturally, you should avoid any exercise when you have an acute, sudden pain, and you should avoid exercise which produces pain or makes an existing pain worse, but the available evidence suggests that, far from causing problems, gentle exercise will help relieve persistent pain.

It does this partly by helping to strengthen muscles which may be weak and partly by providing some distraction. But exercise also has another far more specific pain-suppressing effect. When you exercise your body, messages of command have to travel down from your brain to your spinal cord and eventually to the muscles that you want to move. While those messages are travelling they inhibit the transmission of pain messages going in the opposite direction. Put very simply, the gate through which nerve messages of any sort must pass is so small that it can only allow a certain number of messages to pass through it at any one time; and messages travelling down from the brain to the muscles take precedence over messages trying to travel up from the muscles to the brain.

The other enormous advantage of exercise is, of course, that because it helps you to become mobile it also helps you to become more independent. The more active you become and the more you do, the less restricting your pain will be in other ways.

Pain Control Programme prescription

1. If you're planning to start introducing exercise into your life you must be careful. If you do too much too soon you'll do far more harm than good, and if you stubbornly continue to exercise even though you're in pain you'll damage your body.

You must learn to stop exercising at the very first sign of real pain starting.

Remember, if you always exercise until it hurts then your mind will eventually begin to associate exercise with pain. And unless you're a committed masochist you'll find yourself increasingly reluctant to continue exercising. If your regular exercises don't produce pain but actually make things more comfortable, you'll adopt a much more positive attitude towards exercise in general.

And don't worry if you can't do very much exercise to begin with. Continue exercising and you'll soon find that your pain tolerance levels will go up.

2. Don't rush out and buy roomfuls of expensive exercise equipment. You're unlikely to need any equipment at all but you should certainly wait a while before spending money on gadgets.

3. Apart from taking care not to exercise until you are making your pain worse, there are only two important things you must remember when planning exercise.
a. Don't do anything that your doctor has forbidden. If you are in any doubt then have a word with him before you start and ask him if he has any specific instructions for you. You should be able to get an answer to this question simply by telephoning the surgery at some appropriate time.
b. Don't do any heavy lifting or any labour that involves a great deal of straining.

4. There are two main types of exercise: specific exercise designed to help strengthen parts of your body which are weak, and general exercise intended to improve your general health. Before planning your personal exercise programme

you should decide exactly what you hope to gain by exercising.

5. The best types of general exercise are swimming, walking, dancing and cycling. Of these the type of exercise most suitable for pain sufferers is probably swimming, especially if you can find a pool where the water is reasonably warm. Most people who suffer from back pains or joint troubles find that they can exercise very easily and comfortably in warm water. Jogging and running are not good types of exercise: they tend to aggravate bone and joint problems.

6. There are specific exercises for painful joints. Below I have listed some exercise ideas for particular joints. You should do these exercises as often as you can – remembering that you should always stop exercising if it produces fresh pain or starts to make existing pain noticeably worse.

SHOULDERS
a. Stand facing a wall. Place one hand flat on the wall and by contracting and expanding your fingers make your hand crawl up the wall as far as it will go. See how far you can go. Then try the exercise again later. Measure your daily progress. Do this exercise with each arm in turn.
b. Hold a walking stick in the middle and rotate the stick from side to side.
c. Lie flat on your back on the floor with your arms by your sides. Move your right arm sideways as far as it will go. Then bring it back. Then take it out sideways again. Repeat this with your left arm.
d. Lie flat on your back on the floor. Raise your right arm slowly. Then lower it again. Repeat this with your left arm.
e. Loop a scarf over a door handle and hold one end in each hand. Pull each end of the scarf in turn with a sawing backwards-and-forwards motion.

ELBOWS
a. Lie on your back with your arms by your side, palms down. Then bend your elbow, turning your palm inwards and pointing your fingers towards the ceiling. Next, bring

your palm as close to your shoulder as you can. Take the hand back. Now repeat the exercise with your other arm.
b. Sit as comfortably as you can and simply try bending and straightening your arm as far as you can.

WRISTS AND HANDS
a. Make a fist with your fingers. Then straighten your fingers out as far as you can.
b. Rotate each wrist.
c. Spread out your fingers as far as you can. Then bring the fingers in close together.
d. Wet a cloth and try to wring it dry with both hands.
e. Make a waving movement with your hands, moving them up and down while keeping your forearms stable.
f. Squeeze a tennis ball.
g. Move your thumb across to the base of your little finger.

NECK
a. Move your head round and round.
b. Move your head as far forwards as you can and then as far backwards as you can.

SPINE
a. Lie on your back with your knees bent. Then pull in your tummy muscles as far as they will go.
b. Get into position (a). Then lift your buttocks off the floor.
c. Lie flat on your back with your knees bent and your feet on the floor. Then raise your right knee up to your chest – take it as close as you can get it. Lower your right knee and repeat the exercise with your left knee.
d. Get into position (c). Then try to sit up and touch your knees.
e. Stand with your feet apart and bend sideways, first to the left, then to the right. Try and touch your knees with your hands – one at a time.
f. Stand with your feet apart and try to lean over and touch your toes. It doesn't matter if you can't get anywhere near them: the idea is to get some movement into your spine. Nor does it matter if you bend your knees.

HIPS

a. Lie on your side on your bed. Lift your uppermost leg straight up, away from the lower leg. Do this first on your right side, then on your left.

b. Sit in an upright chair. Try and put your head as near to your knees as possible.

c. Lie on your back with your legs apart. Then slowly try to move your left leg as far away from your right leg as you can. Repeat the exercise with the other leg.

d. Lie flat on your back on the floor (or a bed) and try crossing one leg over the other.

e. Stand upright. Hold on to the back of a chair. Stand on one leg, keeping it straight, and move the other leg round and round. Wave it about. Then repeat the exercise with the other leg.

KNEES

a. Lie flat on your back, lift your legs in the air and pedal an imaginary cycle.

b. Lie on your back. Bend one leg as much as you can, getting your heel close to your buttock. Then straighten it again. Repeat the exercise with the other leg.

c. Sit on the edge of the bed with your legs hanging down. Then straighten one leg. Try lifting the leg as high as you can. Repeat the exercise with the other leg.

ANKLES AND FEET

a. Sit with your feet flat on the floor. Keep your toes on the ground and raise your heels as high as you can.

b. Sit as in position (a). Keep your toes and heel on the ground and try to lift the centre part of your foot off the ground, to make a bridge.

c. Sit with your legs crossed and bend the foot that is in the air as far as it will go. Repeat this exercise with the other foot.

d. Sit as in position (c). Circle your foot round and round, drawing a large, imaginary circle with your big toe. Repeat with the other foot.

Eat Wisely

To reduce your susceptibility to pain you need to keep your body as fit and as healthy as possible. Since you are what you eat, you should obviously take care to ensure that you eat wisely. I suggest that you follow these instructions.

Pain Control Programme prescription

1. If you are overweight you must lose weight. And once you have reached a stable and sensible weight you must not allow yourself to put on excess weight. Every unwanted or unnecessary pound of fat will put extra pressure on your joints, muscles and organs. Many patients who suffer from persistent or recurrent pain could solve their problems permanently simply by losing unnecessary weight. It is certainly true to say that many thousands of individuals who suffer from back trouble could avoid future problems by losing unwanted pounds. (See also page 172.)

Follow these guidelines carefully in order to avoid putting on excess weight.

a. Eat only when you are hungry. Inside your body there is an effective and powerful appetite control centre: follow its needs and you will eat only what your body needs. Ignore it and you will put on weight and stay plump. And remember: stop eating as soon as you no longer feel hungry.

b. Concentrate on your eating. Many people eat while they are reading, working or watching television, and it is difficult to listen to your appetite control centre telling you that you have had enough to eat while you are concentrating on something else.

c. Learn to be more assertive when you are eating. If you continue to allow other people to determine your dietary intake then you will undoubtedly spend your life being overweight. If you let other people decide how much food to put on your plate, how many portions to give you and when you can stop eating, you will end up with a long-term weight problem. If you are to control your weight permanently you must learn to control your own intake of food. Remember that it is the people who insist on you having a second helping who are behaving unreasonably.

d. Be prepared to leave unwanted food on the side of your plate. Many people are reluctant to leave food on their plates or to throw food away. Others eat other people's left-overs too. These habits have to change. Once you have had enough to eat then excess food is a waste – whether you dump it into the bin or dump it into your body. If you choose the latter alternative you'll get fat.

e. Try not to eat late at night – after 7 or 8 p.m. Your body probably won't need the calories and they'll be converted directly into fat. If you feel peckish before you go to bed then have a low-calorie drink.

f. If you eat to cheer yourself up – or to cope with boredom – then find new ways to cope. Treat yourself to a book or a magazine or whatever else you fancy. The amount you spend on unnecessary food is probably high, so your non-fattening treats needn't break the bank.

If you need to *lose* weight follow the guidelines above, but also follow these additional guidelines.

g. Try to trick your body into feeling full when it isn't. Have a low-calorie drink (water, low-calorie lemonade or cola, lemon tea or black coffee, unsweetened or, if you must, with artificial sweetener) half an hour before you eat. This will ensure that your appetite is much reduced. You'll then eat less.

h. Create a sensible weight-loss programme for yourself. If you start off with a long-term plan to lose four stones you will probably lose heart well before you've lost your first stone. The target is too big and too unattainable. Begin with a shorter-term goal – intending to lose, say, ten pounds –

and you will gain your objective far more speedily. The success will give you more confidence and that will boost the chances of your long-term dieting success. You'll think of yourself as a winner.

2. Follow these general eating guidelines.

a. Try to avoid sugar completely. It contains no useful or essential building materials for your body. But it will make you fat, rot your teeth and increase your chances of developing diabetes.

The truth is that you don't need sugar at all. And yet if you regularly put sugar into your drinks then your weekly consumption of sugar could be as high as one pound. Cut your sugar intake in half by using sweeteners instead of sugar and you could, over the course of just one year, save yourself nearly 50,000 calories. That means that in one twelve-month period you could lose fourteen pounds of excess fat simply by using sweeteners instead of sugar.

b. Try to avoid caffeine. It is an addictive and potentially dangerous stimulant which may increase your susceptibility to pain. If you wake up every morning desperate for a cup of coffee then you are probably addicted to caffeine (the same thing is true if you feel a craving for caffeine at other times of the day) and you may well suffer unpleasant side effects, such as headaches, during the withdrawal period.

Remember too that alcohol and nicotine are both powerful and potentially dangerous substances which will interfere with your ability to sleep at night and which may increase your susceptibility to pain.

c. Avoid animal fats such as butter, cream and milk. Use vegetable oil for cooking, and grill rather than fry. Eat no more than two eggs a week. Not only are all fats and oils high in calories, but animal fats in particular increase your likelihood of developing heart disease and high blood pressure.

d. Eat plenty of fresh fruit and vegetables and wholemeal bread.

Music – the Soothing Pain Killer

The Indians were probably the first to recognize the value of music therapy. Four thousand years ago Hindu doctors used to play soothing gentle music while surgeons were operating. They used to play music in the wards too. They discovered that music helped people to relax and get better quicker.

Only in the last few years, however, have we re-learnt the truth about the healing power of music. It has long been known that music can be soothing and relaxing, and can cheer people up when they are sad, and calm them when they are anxious or over-excited. But it is only quite recently that we have realized how much it can help people move more easily when they are stiff or uncomfortable, can bring back happy memories to people who are troubled by depression and despair and, of course, can help relieve pain.

In one of the most remarkable experiments conducted to show the pain-relieving value of music Drs M. Borzecki and K. Zakrzewski of the Pain Clinic at the Warsaw Academy of Medicine used music to help seventeen patients suffering from backache, headaches and trigeminal neuralgia. They found that music had an extremely valuable effect on their patients and helped to control even quite savage pains.

Pain Control Programme prescription

1. Collect a library of the cassettes, tapes or records which you find most soothing. Learn to use the music you have chosen as often as possible. The type of music you choose will depend, of course, upon your personal tastes and prefer-ences. Some people find classical music most relaxing. Others

prefer hard rock music. Many seem to find soothing, traditional ballads most calming.

2. A portable cassette recorder with a pair of headphones will enable you to enjoy your favourite music wherever you are, without annoying your neighbours. You are also likely to find it easier to 'lose' yourself in your music if you use headphones.

3. Don't forget that you can benefit by playing music as well as listening to it. The piano and the guitar seem to be the two instruments most likely to prove soothing.

Learn to Relax Your Body

Pain is your body's way of telling you to stop whatever it is that you are doing, an early warning signal designed to tell your brain that your body is at risk. Inevitably, therefore, when you are in pain your body will respond in exactly the same way that it will respond to stress or danger. Your heart will beat faster, your rate of breathing will go up and your muscles will become tense. All these developments are designed to help you cope more effectively with the danger that your body assumes is threatening you.

If the pain is a short-lived event the changes which take place help you avoid further injury. If you are bitten on the leg by a dog then your body's responses to the pain (and the accompanying fear) will be to prepare your body for instant action. You will, therefore, be better able to escape from the dog and avoid being bitten again. You'll be able to run quickly or climb a tree and get out of the dog's way. Your tensed muscles will have helped you.

If, however, your pain is a long-term problem the increased tension in your muscles is not likely to help you at all. Having tense muscles won't help you escape from a back problem or an inflamed joint.

In fact, the tensing of your muscles is very likely to make things far worse by putting extra pressure on your bones and joints. This is exactly what happens to a lot of people when they are in pain. Their tensed muscles put them under a tremendous amount of muscular pressure and result in existing symptoms getting worse and new symptoms, such as headaches, developing.

Pain Control Programme prescription

If you feel that your muscles really become tense when you are in pain then you will benefit enormously from following the advice below.

1. Take very slow, deep breaths. Pain will usually make you breathe unusually quickly, which will result in your blood not being properly oxygenated. This in turn can lead to all sorts of additional muscle pains and cramps. Deliberately breathe as slowly and as deeply as you possibly can.

2. Learn to relax the muscles throughout your body by following this simple regimen. First, lie down somewhere quiet and comfortable.
a. Clench your left hand as tightly as you can, making a fist with the fingers. Do it well and you will see the knuckles go white. If you now let your fist unfold you will feel the muscles relax. When your hand was clenched the muscles were tensed; unfolded the same muscles are relaxed. This is what you must do with the other muscle groups of your body.
b. Bend your left arm and try to make your left biceps muscle stand out as much as you can. Then relax it and let the muscles ease. Let your arm lie loosely by your side and ignore it.
c. Relax your right hand in the same way.
d. Relax your right biceps muscle in the same way.
e. Tighten the muscles in your left foot. Curl your toes. When the foot feels as tense as you can make it, let it relax.
f. Tense the muscles of your left calf. If you reach down you can feel the muscles at the back of your leg firm up as you tense them. Bend your foot towards you to help tighten up the muscles. Then let the muscles relax.
g. Straighten your leg and point your foot away from you. You will feel the muscles on the front of your thigh tighten up; they should be firm right up to the top of your leg. Now relax the muscles.
h. Relax your right foot.
i. Relax your right lower leg.

j. Relax your right thigh.

k. Lift yourself up by tightening up your buttock muscles. You will be able to lift your body upwards by an inch or so. Then let your muscles fall loose again.

l. Tense and contract your abdominal muscles. Try to pull your abdominal wall as far in as possible. Then let go and allow your waist to reach its maximum circumference.

m. Tighten the muscles of your chest. Take a big, deep breath in and strain to hold it for as long as possible. Then let go.

n. Push your shoulders backwards as far as they will go, then bring them forward and inwards. Finally shrug them as high as you can. Keep your head perfectly still and try to touch your ears with your shoulders. It will probably be impossible, but try anyway. Then let your shoulders relax and ease.

o. Next tighten up the muscles of your back. Try to make yourself as tall as you can. Then let the muscles relax.

p. The muscles of the neck are next. Lift your head forwards and pull at the muscles at the back of your neck. Turn your head first one way and then the other. Push your head backwards with as much force as you can. Then let the muscles of your neck relax. Move your head around and make sure that the neck muscles are completely loose and easy.

q. Move your eyebrows upwards and then pull them down as far as they will go. Do this several times, making sure that you can feel the muscles tightening both when you move the eyebrows up and when you pull them down. Then let them relax.

r. Screw up your eyes as tightly as you can. Pretend that someone is trying to force your eyes open. Keep them shut tightly. Then, keeping your eyelids closed, let them relax.

s. Move your lower jaw around. Grit your teeth. Wrinkle your nose. Smile as wide as you can showing as many teeth as you can. Now let all these facial muscles relax.

t. Push your tongue out as far as it will go, push it firmly against the bottom of your mouth and the top of your mouth and then let it lie relaxed and easy inside your mouth.

Control Your Stress

The human body was originally designed for a world full of physical threats and dangers. Consequently our bodies respond to fear in a very simple and straightforward physical way: our hearts beat faster, our blood pressure goes up and our muscles tighten. Our bodies are, in general, put on alert so that we can run faster, climb higher and fight better.

In a world full of sabre-toothed tigers and the like, such responses were essential for survival. If Stone Age man came out of his cave and found himself face to face with a man-eating bear without being more or less instantly prepared for action, he wouldn't have lasted long.

Unfortunately, of course, our problems these days aren't quite so simple or straightforward. Instead of finding ourselves face to face with a sabre-toothed tiger, a pack of hungry wolves or an angry bear we are far more likely to find ourselves having to face unemployment, big gas bills or officious policemen. None of these modern problems can be dealt with by a faster heart rate, a higher blood pressure or tense muscles. Those natural physiological responses won't help you cope more effectively.

And yet, when your body thinks that it is in a dangerous situation, it continues to respond in that same old-fashioned way. The longer you worry about unemployment, gas bills and the other thousand and one fears and irritations of twentieth-century life, the longer your body will stay on alert. Faced with a threat of any kind, your body continues to respond in the only way it knows how: by preparing for physical action.

The problem is that we have changed our world far faster than our bodies have been able to adapt. At no other time in the history of the world has there been such a constant progression of ideas. Never before have living conditions, attitudes and fashions changed so rapidly. Our world has been transformed. But our bodies are much the same as they were many thousands of years ago. It takes hundreds of thousands of years for the human body to adapt and we have changed our civilization far too quickly for our own good. Our bodies still respond to threats in the same way that they would have responded thousands of years ago. But today our responses are sadly inappropriate.

Often your body's natural responses to anxiety and stress cause illness and distress. In particular there is now a strong and well-established relationship between anxiety, stress and pressure and the development of pain.

When you get home at the end of the day carrying with you a thousand separate worries, and you arrive to find your world there packed with even more worries and anxieties, it is hardly surprising that you end up with a persistent headache, a recurrent backache or a terrible griping pain in your abdomen.

Fears, stresses and anxieties are cumulative. You worry about whether or not your job is going to be safe next year. Your body responds by tensing your muscles a little, believing that since you are worried a physical response must be appropriate. As far as your body is concerned, you are in danger. Then you worry about the fact that the mortgage rate is supposed to be going up. Your body responds again by increasing the muscle tension around your body. Next you start worrying about your daughter's health. Or the fact that the car is making a funny noise. Or the rumour that a foreign company may buy your employer's company and make you redundant. Or the possibility that the council will be building a dual carriageway at the bottom of your garden. Or the fact that your dahlias don't look well. And each time you introduce new worry to your life your blood pressure rises a little higher and your muscles become more and more tensed.

'What, me?' you say, when the doctor asks you if you've been under any stress lately. 'No, nothing in particular.'

There are two quite different ways in which you can help yourself if you suspect that stress or pressure could be producing your pain or simply making it worse.

First, since the type of pain most commonly produced by anxiety and pressure is usually caused by muscle tension, you can learn to help yourself by deliberately learning how to relax your muscles and your mind. If you relax your muscles you'll be able to ease the tension in your body and reduce the extent of your pain. If you relax your mind you'll be able to stop your muscles getting tense at all. These two techniques are discussed on pages 145ff. and 80ff. of my Pain Control Programme.

Second, if stress and pressure are helping to cause your pain you can help yourself by learning how to reduce your exposure and your susceptibility to stress and pressure.

The section which follows contains advice on how best you can control your stress.

Pain Control Programme prescription

1. You must control your exposure to stress by limiting the things that you do. If you feel that you are constantly under pressure then try to reduce some of your commitments. So, for example, if you have a hectic business life and a busy home life then you should take care to ensure that you do not add extra stress to your life by spending your evenings working on committees or in local politics.

Try to make sure that you have at least half a day a week when you have no outside commitments and you can simply relax and take things easy.

If your life is already filled with stresses and pressures then take up a peaceful, low-pressure hobby such as fishing or gardening. Don't make the mistake of allowing stress and pressure to enter your leisure time. Too many people who take up sports or games in order to help them relax end up taking their hobby far too seriously. Fishing won't help your muscles relax if you spend your days desperately trying to catch the world's biggest salmon or trying to get into the British Angling Team.

2. Learn to recognize the early warning signs that tell you when the pressure is beginning to damage your body. Most of us have a weak point. When the pressure is getting too much we develop a physical or mental symptom that should act as a trigger sign telling us that we are doing too much and that we need to pull back a little.

These early warning signs show that you are beginning to suffer real damage as a result of the stress to which you are exposed. Your stress threshold has been breached, and if you don't take some fairly rapid action your problems will merely increase.

Any physical or mental sign or symptom that becomes more apparent when you have been under pressure is an early warning sign. But as a guide look through the following list – it includes some of the commonest physical and mental warning signs.

Headache
Skin rash
Palpitations
Chest pains
Diarrhoea
Indigestion or stomach pains
Tiredness
Wheezing
Irritability
Reduced willpower
Intolerance of noise
Inability to feel relaxed
Inability to concentrate
Poor memory
Crying a lot
Inability to finish tasks you have started
Over-reacting to little things
Impulsive behaviour

Whether or not it is on this list, you must learn to look out for your early warning sign. When it becomes clear that your early warning sign has been triggered then you must take some action: you need to relax, pull back a little and take time out. If you don't, you will very likely develop serious pains before too long.

3. If you are going to control the amount of stress in your life (and the effect that stress has on your health) you must learn to organize yourself properly. People who don't plan ahead often end up in a terrible mess. If you set off to do your shopping and you don't take a list with you, the chances are that when you get back home you'll have suddenly remembered several items that you really wanted to buy. You'll either have to do without or make a second journey back to the shops again. If you set off on a long motoring journey and you fail to fill up with petrol, oil, air and water then the chances are that you'll break down somewhere en route. If you sit down and send out Christmas cards without having a list by your side then before you're half way through the task you'll be in a terrible mess.

Bad organization and failing to plan ahead properly can often lead to increased stress loads, to pressure and to the development of severe and troublesome pains.

To avoid these extra and unnecessary stresses I suggest that you keep a notebook and a pencil by your side at all times. Write down any problems that seem significant or that have to be remembered. When they're written down on paper many problems seem far less significant.

If you're planning some special event, such as a house move or a large celebration, keep a special master plan to help you keep things running smoothly. List everything that needs to be done and mark off the dates by which each problem has to be solved. You can cut your worry and anxiety (and unwanted muscle pains) enormously by doing this. Keeping lists and using them isn't a sign of mental weakness, it's a sign of mental strength.

And when you've got a really difficult problem to solve write down all the alternative solutions in your notebook. Keep your notebook handy and add new solutions as they occur to you. Keep your notebook by your bedside, because good ideas often pop into your head last thing at night just when you're about to go to sleep. Take your notebook into the bathroom with you too. Then, when you need to make a decision, look down your list and select the best possible solution. You'll probably find that by this time one particular answer stands out.

Treat Your Pain Aggressively

If you suffer from pain a good deal you will probably find that before long your pain begins to run your life and to dominate your relationships with other people. Because most people are naturally sympathetic towards any individual in discomfort friends, relatives and even strangers will tend to treat you rather specially.

It will start innocently enough, with those around you making a fuss of you and insisting that you avoid all sorts of ordinary responsibilities and duties. People will want to adjust your pillows, pass you the newspaper, make you a drink, change the television channel for you and generally turn you into a complete invalid. Your friends and relatives will behave in this way out of kindness, of course, but they will be teaching you to behave in a very special sort of way. They will be teaching you to behave in the way that they expect a patient in pain to behave. They will assume that your pain prevents you from living a normal life and they will encourage you to use your pain as an excuse. You will receive sympathy, attention and respect. You'll be able to avoid unpleasant confrontations and unsatisfying chores. You'll be allowed to avoid work, gardening, housework and (if you want to) even sex because of your pain.

To begin with your relatives and friends will be inspired by love and sympathy. They will want to see you get better and they will hope that by treating you in this way they will be able to help you get better quicker while at the same time avoiding unnecessary discomfort.

But, if your pain persists, then things will slowly but inevitably change.

However much your friends and relatives may love you,

they will begin to lose patience. They will feel inadequate because, despite all their efforts, your pain will not have disappeared. Indeed, because you've been resting, your pain will have probably been getting worse. They will have done everything they can to help you but you won't have improved. They won't know what else they can do. They'll lose heart, they'll feel embarrassed and they'll begin to feel faintly irritated. They will want to help you but, because your pain has continued, they'll feel that there must be something else that they could have done. They will feel guilty, they won't like feeling guilty and they won't know why they feel guilty; and their visits will probably become less and less frequent.

Meanwhile, you'll probably wonder exactly what is going on. Your friends and relatives won't visit quite so often. They won't be quite so patient or supportive. And you won't know why.

Even more important, the behavioural patterns you'll have been encouraged to adopt will have made it difficult for you to break free. Because you'll have been treated as an invalid, and encouraged to think of yourself as an invalid, you will live like an invalid. The longer you've been bed- or chair-bound, the more difficult you will find physical movement. You won't want to get up or go out. Your life will revolve around your pain. You will be physically weak and your pain will be more and more intolerable. Pill-taking will have probably become a habit that you will be reluctant to break.

Pain Control Programme prescription

You can ensure that your pain does not take over your life by taking a much more aggressive attitude towards both your illness and your pain. And you can do this whether your pain is a fairly recent one or one that has been present for some time. It is, however, vitally important to remember that you are the only person who can take this aggressive approach to your own pain. Your relatives and friends will be driven by sympathy, compassion and love. Their natural response will be to encourage you to give in to your pain.

You must take the initiative and ensure that your pain does not get the chance to run your life.

There are several ways in which you can do this.

1. Responding to pain in a passive way brings a lot of rewards. If you stay in bed all day you'll feel comfortable and warm and people will know that you are in pain. They will treat you with extra care and respect. Getting up and going out will require a tremendous amount of determination. So try to give yourself as many incentives as possible to live as normal a life as you can. Don't just plan on getting up for the sake of getting up. Plan a trip to the cinema, to the pub, to the shops or to see a friend. You need to *want* to get up and go out.

2. Try to take an active, positive role in your own treatment. Try to be as positive as you can about the future. Try to regard your illness as an enemy that can be conquered. Learn as much as you can about what is causing your pain and what makes it worse. If you do what you can to control your own destiny and make a genuine effort to take a positive and aggressive part in your own treatment and future, you will benefit enormously. By remaining active and determined you will reduce the level of pain. And by remaining positive you will weaken your illness and strengthen yourself.

3. Remember that your doctor is human too. He may not understand the importance of the relationship between the mind and the body. Medical students are taught to regard psychiatry and medicine as two quite different disciplines. Your doctor is unlikely to have been taught that the two are in fact closely interlinked. Moreover, because your doctor is human he will feel guilty and inadequate because he has been unable to cure your pain. He will expect to be able to cure you. He will probably find his own failure difficult to accept.

I am not suggesting that you should lie to your doctor about the amount of pain you're suffering. But try not to let your doctor turn you into an invalid. Ask him if you can get up and go out. Ask him to tell you what you must not do.

And do take care not to turn your pain into a challenge for your doctor. An astonishing number of people turn up at their doctors saying things like 'I've been to six doctors and none of them could help me. I don't expect you'll be able to help me either.' If you start off with that sort of negative attitude then you can be certain of two things: your doctor will not be able to help you and your pain will continue unabated.

4. Talk to your friends and relatives and encourage them to offer you support and encouragement, not just when you are sick and in pain and incapacitated but also when you are fighting your pain and struggling to cope with it. If they offer you sympathy, love and affection only when you are immobilized by pain or in tears then you will eventually learn to associate pain with love. And when your mind craves love your body will respond by producing pain. Explain to your relatives and friends that although you need their support and love when you are in pain, you also need their support and love when you are fighting your pain. If they help you in this way then your mind will learn to respond to this new relationship: you will expect to be loved when you fight your pain. And there can be no greater incentive than that.

5. Be blunt with yourself. Ask yourself what benefits you get from your pain. And try to ensure that wherever possible you break the link between pain and benefit.

Know How to Measure Your Pain

It is impossible to measure pain objectively. There are so many different factors involved that it is impossible for you to compare the pain you get in your back with the pain your neighbour gets in her womb. It's quite impossible for you to compare the pains you get in your chest with the headaches which cripple your father.

But you can measure variations in a particular pain. You can tell whether or not a specific pain is getting better or worse. And that can be extremely useful: if you can tell how your pain is changing then you can judge the effectiveness of the different types of treatment that you may be trying.

Pain Control Programme prescription

1. One of the simplest ways of measuring pain is to use an ordinary school ruler. The left-hand end of the ruler marks complete freedom from pain. The right-hand end of the ruler marks the worst pain that you can possibly imagine. Simply look carefully at the ruler and decide just where on that scale your pain should be measured. And then make a note of the reading you've taken. On subsequent occasions you simply look at your ruler again and make a fresh assessment. You can then measure whether your pain seems to be getting worse, getting better or staying the same.

2. Another simple but effective technique is to record your pain level according to this simple chart:
0 = no pain
1 = mild pain

2 = moderate pain
3 = severe pain
4 = intolerable pain
At approximately the same time each day make a note of how you feel, recording your pain as 0, ½, 1, 1½, 2, 2½, 3, 3½, or 4.

3. A more sophisticated technique is to look through the list of words which follow and pick out the four which you think describe your current pain most accurately.

sore (1)
dull (1)
tender (1)
annoying (1)
troublesome (1)
uncomfortable (1)
tiring (2)
hurting (2)
heavy (2)
distressing (2)
miserable (2)
sickening (2)
exhausting (3)
frightful (3)
wretched (3)
intense (3)
horrible (3)
punishing (3)
terrifying (4)
vicious (4)
killing (4)
unbearable (4)
excruciating (4)
intolerable (4)

Add up the numbers that follow each of the words you have chosen. The total is your 'pain score'.

On subsequent occasions simply look through the list again and repeat the procedure, comparing your total score with previous total scores.

Conclusion

The traditional medical approach to the treatment of pain concentrates very much on the purely physical aspects of the problem. Doctors are taught that they must deal with pain by using interventionist remedies such as drugs or surgery.

By using my Pain Control Programme you will be able to deal with your pain in a far more effective and far safer way. Read through my Programme carefully, select those elements which seem most suitable and acceptable, and then use them to create your own personal pain control programme. You can, of course, use any of these techniques together with whatever treatments you and your doctor may consider appropriate.

Finally, do remember that I do not claim that my Programme will cure your pain permanently. I do, however, claim that my Pain Control Programme will reduce the amount of pain you suffer, help you reduce your dependence on drugs, and improve the quality of your life.

APPENDIX

Practical Pain Control

Introduction

My Pain Control Programme can be used to help you deal with any type of recurrent or persistent pain. The sections on the following pages are intended to provide examples of the ways in which you can put the Programme into practice.

Arthritis

Few diseases affect as many people as arthritis, and few cause as much pain and disablement. In Western countries one in every five adults suffers from arthritis. In Britain, for example, there are said to be eight million arthritics.

Although few diseases are as common as arthritis, few are the subject of so many myths, misconceptions and misunderstandings. The main myth is that there is any such thing as a single disease called 'arthritis' or 'rheumatism'. The truth is that these terms are about as useful and specific as the word 'infection'; and just as there are over 100 different types of infection so there are over 100 different types of arthritis and rheumatism. The words arthritis and rheumatism are simply used to describe diseases which damage joints and the tissues around them.

There are nearly 200 different joints in the human body. Each joint consists of two opposing bones, each being capped with a layer of white, smooth, gristly cartilage, enclosed within a capsule and washed in an essential lubricating (synovial) fluid. Tendons attached to the bones help hold the joint in place. Joints enable us to move, to absorb sudden shocks and to walk and run. They can repair themselves when they are injured or damaged, and they can replenish their own supplies of synovial fluid.

Unfortunately, like every other part of the human body, joints can become diseased. There are well over 100 different joint diseases which have been identified. There are probably many more still unidentified.

Diseases which affect joints – arthritic diseases – fall into six basic categories.

First, there are the inflammatory joint disorders in which

the synovial membrane (which is responsible for producing the synovial fluid) becomes red, thick and swollen, resulting in the development of a hot, red, painful, swollen joint. If the disease is uncontrolled the joint will eventually be destroyed. Rheumatoid arthritis is the commonest disease in this category. It usually involves the smaller joints, particularly those in the hands and wrists, and mainly affects men and women between the ages of twenty-five and fifty. The disease affects about three times as many women as men. Just what causes rheumatoid arthritis is still something of a mystery but the symptoms are well known and include pain, tenderness, and swelling and stiffness of the affected joints.

Second, and also very common, is osteoarthritis, a condition which is an almost inevitable result of growing old and which commonly seems to strike between the ages of fifty and sixty, probably affecting slightly more women than men. Osteoarthritis develops as the cartilage which normally protects bone from rubbing on bone is gradually worn away. Excessive wear and tear and damage to a joint can all result in the development of osteoarthritis, but the condition can be inherited; being overweight is another major contributory factor.

The joints most commonly affected by osteoarthritis include the knees, hips, spine, hands and feet. The initial symptoms usually involve aching, stiffness, difficulty in moving and some deformity.

The third-commonest type of arthritis is ankylosing spondylitis; again, this is a rather different type of joint problem. Like rheumatoid arthritis it is believed to be an inflammatory disease, but in this case the inflammation occurs where the ligaments and tendons join the bones. Ankylosing spondylitis usually involves the joints of the spine, but sometimes affects the larger joints of the body. It is a condition that affects more men than women; in particular, it seems to affect men between the ages of fifteen and twenty-five. The symptoms of the condition include pain and stiffness in the back, hips and shoulders, usually worse in the mornings and after rest.

In the fourth type of joint disease the problems are caused by the development of crystals inside the joint. The best-known disease in this category is gout, where pain is caused by the information of uric acid crystals in the joint spaces. Any joint can be affected by gout, but the big toes are the ones most commonly involved. The ankles, knees, wrists, elbows and fingers are also common sites. Gout affects far more men than women (in a ratio of fifteen to one), usually affecting men between the ages of thirty-five and sixty. The initial symptom is a very sudden onset of severe pain in a joint, which will usually be swollen and bluish red. There may be a moderate fever too, but the symptoms will come and go quite unexpectedly.

The fifth category of arthritic diseases include those disorders that develop when organisms such as bacteria or viruses get into a joint.

The sixth type of arthritis doesn't involve bones or joints at all, but affects the muscles which surround a joint. When muscles are strained or inflamed the resulting symptoms can be very similar to some types of true arthritis and although these disorders are not, strictly speaking, joint problems they are often described as being types of arthritis.

Despite the fact that that all these disorders are extremely common, arthritics are not, I fear, particularly well looked after by the medical profession. One problem is undoubtedly the fact that doctors are taught very little about arthritis. Apart from the explanation that there is no cure for arthritis and it is not, therefore, a particularly satisfying disease to treat, I can't imagine why this should be. The fact remains, however, that in 1981 the Arthritis and Rheumatism Council in Britain complained that millions of sufferers from arthritis and rheumatism experience needless pain simply because doctors don't know enough about how to treat the disease. They reported that in a third of British medical schools there is very little training given to medical students in the treatment of arthritis; on average the time allocated to rheumatology in a medical school course is a mere thirty-six hours.

The single commonest symptom endured by patients suffering from arthritic disorders is undoubtedly pain. In an inflamed or damaged joint there is, it seems, a change in the way that the nerves which carry messages from the joint respond to pressures and strains. It seems that relatively small changes of pressure can produce great surges of pain in an arthritic joint.

The standard medical treatment for arthritis involves drugs. Most of the major international drug companies now make a wide range of products specially designed to help alleviate the pain of arthritis. Most of these products are variations on the traditional 'aspirin' theme; but in fact most experts agree that the single most useful drug for the treatment of arthritis and the alleviation of the symptoms associated with arthritis, is ordinary soluble aspirin.

Pain Control Programme in practice

Any or all of the elements of my Pain Control Programme may relieve the pain of your arthritis. For example:

1. When the pain of arthritis is at its worst you should rest. But when the acute pain is over then you should exercise your joints as much as possible. Movement helps to ensure that the joints are not allowed to become stiff. Swimming in warm water is the best form of exercise available. Walking is also useful, but do try to walk on soft ground rather than hard roads or pavements: the shocks produced by walking (or even worse, jogging) on hard ground can result in a considerable amount of joint damage.

2. The TENS device described on pages 120–25 is known to be extremely useful in the treatment of arthritic pains. A group of doctors in Glasgow have done research with thirty patients suffering from painful, osteoarthritic knees. The patients found that TENS was two and a half times as effective as paracetamol as a pain reliever. A second report from Montreal has shown that patients with muscular aches and pains also benefit from using TENS; while a third report, this time from Cambridge, has shown that TENS has a very useful pain-relieving effect on shoulder pains.

3. Learning how to relax your mind and your body can have a very useful effect on pain of the type produced by arthritis.

A report published in 1981 by Jeanne Achterberg of the University of Texas Health Science Center in Dallas and Phillip McGraw and G. Frank Lawlis of North Texas State University showed that when twenty-four patients were taught how to relax they suffered considerably less pain. Since it has been known for some time that stress and tension can make arthritis worse, it is reassuring to know that relaxation can make it better.

4. If you suffer from arthritis, every extra pound of weight you carry will make your arthritis worse. If you don't suffer from arthritis, every extra pound of weight you carry will increase your chances of developing arthritis. You can reduce the amount of stress on, and therefore pain in, your joints by reducing your weight.

5. If you suffer from arthritis you should make every effort to keep your mind, as well as your body, as busy as possible. There is now plenty of evidence to show that the more active you are the more likely it is that your arthritis will be kept under control. Unless you are suffering from acute pain do not stay in bed or even in your house. You should do everything you can to keep yourself occupied with work or with captivating leisure activities.

6. It has been shown that laughter has a very useful and positive effect on inflammatory arthritic conditions. The more you can laugh, the less pain you will have.

Backache

According to a report published in the medical journal *Update* in November 1985, over 23 million Britons suffer from back pain in any one year. That is well over half the adult population. In another survey it was found that between one-quarter and one-third of all the individuals interviewed claimed to have experienced back pain in the two weeks prior to the interview. The majority of back pain sufferers are between thirty-five and fifty-five years old.

The pain and the personal agony caused by all this backache is phenomenal, but impossible to estimate in any measurable terms. Far easier to estimate is the financial cost of all this sickness. It has been computed that back pain causes more time off work than any other single complaint or cause. Nearly 1 per cent of the population have time off work each year through back pain. Twenty million working days are lost every year through back pain and on any one working day there are some 80,000 people off work with backache. Back pain costs Britain something like £1.5 billion pounds a year – that's equivalent to twelve months' output of a medium-sized town.

Over recent years doctors have made all sorts of attempts to work out just why we suffer so much from backache. And although there is much confusion and controversy over exactly what happens, there is some agreement about the problem in general terms. In four out of every five cases of back pain doctors never find out what has caused the pain. In the majority of patients there are no physical abnormalities to be found – even on X-ray examination.

It seems that back pain first became a real problem when we started standing up and walking around erect, rather than on all fours. If you believe in the Creation you will have to put the blame on our Maker. If you believe in evolution you'll have to accept that we have not yet evolved far enough to make standing up physiologically sound.

Although the thirty-three vertebrae, the small bones which make up the spine, fit neatly on top of one another they were never really designed for an upright posture. The spine is strong enough to withstand pressures of several hundred pounds, and is so flexible that it can be bent to form two-thirds of a circle, but the intricate system of muscles, tendons and ligaments which keep the whole thing together can easily be damaged or disrupted in all sorts of ways. The spine acts as a scaffolding for the whole of the body, with skull, ribs, pelvis and limbs all attached to it. Through its middle runs the extremely delicate spinal cord, so that even a relatively slight physical abnormality can result in many kinds of awful pain.

Because they recognize that doctors can do little to help back pain, only about 10 per cent of back pain sufferers bother to consult their family doctor. And only rarely are the patients who do see doctors actually helped by medical treatment. Fewer than one in every 1,000 people with back pain need surgery; even fewer than that benefit from it.

In a way, that is perhaps not all that surprising. After all, back specialists admit that something like 80 per cent of all back pain problems aren't caused by physical problems at all but by stress and worry. Most people will be able to gain far more from my Pain Control Programme than from medical treatment.

Pain Control Programme in practice

Any or all of the elements of my Pain Control Programme may relieve your back pain. For example:

1. If you have acute pain in your back then you must rest – and rest in bed until the pain has eased. In a controlled clinical trial involving a group of soldiers with back pain it was shown that the soldiers who rested in bed returned to

their normal duties in half the time taken by the soldiers who didn't. When resting you must make sure that you do exactly that. For most people that means staying in bed taking the pressure off your back by lying flat, but in natural and comfortable positions. Many ailments can be helped while you rest sitting with a book or helping with the washing up, but acute backache needs proper bed rest.

2. According to a series of studies conducted by Surrey University's Department of Human Biology, an estimated 20,000 nurses working in National Health Service hospitals in Britain suffer from back pain ever year. In four out of five cases the pain is caused by injuries the nurses have sustained while lifting or moving patients.

When lifting or picking things up you should take care not to bend from the waist. You should bend at the knees and keep your back as straight as possible. It may feel natural to lift by bending your back, but you'll put a tremendous amount of strain on your back muscles if you do so.

It isn't just lifting that causes back pain. In recent years it has become clear that many cases of backache develop because patients do not understand the ways in which their backs can most easily be damaged. One of the most important aspects of my Pain Control Programme is that you should understand your illness, and thus know how to avoid exacerbating an existing problem.

Below I have listed some simple advice intended to help you avoid putting your back under unnecessary pressure.

a. Make sure that your bed is not contributing to your problem. Your bed should have a firm mattress or you should sleep with a wooden board between the mattress and the springs. You should sleep on your side with your knees bent slightly. Sleeping on your stomach increases the likelihood of back pain developing.

b. Avoid high-heeled shoes whenever possible. They throw the spine out of line and can lead to long-term pain problems.

c. Car seats are notoriously troublesome. If you can adjust your car seat, do so every half hour or so on long journeys. Put a cushion at the base of your spine. And stop your car regularly and walk around for a few minutes. Do a few stretching and bending exercises too.

d. Prolonged standing in one position puts a tremendous strain on the back. If you're at a party, keep circulating round the room. If you're drinking at a bar, lean first on one elbow and then on the other elbow.

e. Heavy shoulder bags are bad for your spine unless you move them from one side to the other at regular intervals.

f. If you spend a lot of time sitting and working at a desk make sure that your desk and chair are at the correct relative heights. Make sure that your desk is well lit. Get up and stretch your back muscles regularly.

3. Exercise will help strengthen your back and tone up your muscles in general. Swimming and walking are particularly suitable general exercises. Do remember that jogging on hard surfaces is very bad for your back and is a common cause of back pain.

You should also do exercises specifically designed to strengthen the muscles that support your spine (see page 138).

4. A good massage can help relieve stiffness in the back muscles and prevent back pain developing. Remember not to do anything that produces pain. Read pages 114ff. for more specific details. Do not manipulate or put pressure on the spine itself.

5. Heat helps ease back pain. You can try a hot-water bottle or an electric heating pad, but the most effective way to apply heat to your back is to lie in a warm bath for twenty minutes or half an hour.

6. Learn to relax properly. Stress and tension are the commonest causes of back pain. You can deal with your back pain and help prevent your pain returning by learning how to relax your mind and how to deal with stress.

7. If you are overweight you must diet. Ten pounds of excess weight carried on your abdomen is equivalent to a pressure

of 100 pounds of additional weight inside your spine. As your abdomen gets bigger so your buttocks are pushed out to balance the weight increase and so your spine gets pushed out of shape. That is why back pain is so common among pregnant women.

8. TENS has been shown to help many back pain patients. And yet remarkably few doctors realize that TENS devices are now readily available. I recently read a new book on the subject of back pain in which TENS was mentioned on two lines merely as a new and possibly promising therapy. There is more evidence to prove the value of TENS than there ever has been to prove the value of most of the drugs doctors prescribe so freely.

9. You should buy a rocking chair. The backward and forward movement will help relieve your pain considerably by stimulating your nerves to produce impulses which will then block pain impulses. If doctors handed out free rocking chairs to their back pain patients the amount of money saved on drugs would be tremendous.

10. Ice often helps patients suffering from back pain. The available evidence suggests that ice treatment is particularly suitable for patients suffering from low back pain.

Cancer Pain

Cancer is a strange disease: very often it can develop for some time without producing any pain. Cancer cells are made up of almost all the same chemical components as normal body cells and the human body's defence mechanisms don't recognize cancer cells as being foreign, or indeed anything to worry about. If a peanut goes down into your lung then you'll cough and splutter and end up in quite a lot of pain. But a lung cancer can develop inside your lung and grow to the size of a grapefruit without causing any symptoms at all.

When cancer pain does develop it is usually because the cancer has grown to such a size that it is pressing on some internal structure or interfering in some way with the functioning of the body. So, for example, if a cancer starts pressing on a nerve then the nerve may start transmitting pain messages to the brain.

Just how many cancer patients do suffer from pain is not known. Kathleen Foley, chief of the pain service at the Memorial Sloan Kettering Cancer Center in New York, suggests that only about one-third of cancer patients develop severe pain. The World Health Organization has suggested an estimate of 50 per cent. Dr A. G. Larson, consultant anaesthetist for Portsmouth District Hospitals has reported that 75 per cent of cancer patients develop pain.

To a large extent, however, the question of how many patients suffer pain is academic. It is far more important to be able to find out how many cancer patients have pain that is difficult or impossible to relieve with drugs or other treatments. And here there are figures available. Studies carried out in hospitals and hospices in both the United Kingdom and the United States of America suggest that about 25 per cent of all cancer patients die with severe and unrelieved pain.

Obviously, many patients who suffer from cancer need treatment with morphine. As I have pointed out on page 56, when morphine is given it is important that it is given in large enough doses. When morphine is being used as a pain reliever there is never any need to worry about side effects or patients becoming addicted.

But it is also important to remember that morphine is nothing more than a drug which imitates internally-produced pain relieving hormones, the endorphins. And it must also be borne in mind that the production of these pain-relieving hormones can be stimulated by many of the techniques described in my Pain Control Programme.

Pain Control Programme in practice

Any or all of the elements of my Pain Control Programme may relieve cancer pain. For example:

1. Imagery is one of the most effective ways of dealing with pain, but it is also an extremely effective way of dealing with cancer. And, of course, it's much more sensible to use imagery to deal with the cause rather than the symptoms. So I suggest that cancer patients who want to use this technique use it to attack their cancer.

Some of the most impressive results in this field have come from Dr Carl Simonton and his wife in America. For a number of years now they have been teaching patients how to cope with cancer by using their imaginations. In the first years of their work the Simontons have found that their patients have lived on average more than a year longer than patients who were not encouraged to use their minds to help fight their disease.

Other evidence illustrating the effectiveness of imagery techniques is coming in all the time.

In the *Daily Mail* in June 1985 Jill Ireland, the actress wife of Hollywood tough guy star Charles Bronson, described how she had used imagery techniques to help her fight cancer: 'I began visualising cancer cells, then telling myself that cancer is a weak disease, composed of weak, confused, deformed cells . . . I visualised my white blood cells. I imagined them as piranha fish. They poured into the areas where the cancer cells were and destroyed them and I visualised them going around quietly and competently doing their job, taking care of my body and, if they saw any cancer cells, they destroyed them.'

You can, of course, adapt this type of imagery technique to suit your own personal imagination. If you want, think of your cancer cells as being bandits or red Indians, or space monsters or robbers. And think of your body's defences, the good white blood cells, disguised as heroes, cowboys, spacemen or policemen. Imagine your body's defences tearing round your body and destroying the frightened cancer cells.

2. Learn to assert yourself.

If the doctors and nurses who are looking after you won't tell you things that you feel you want to know, then make a fuss and a nuisance of yourself until they answer your questions. It is important that you know what is going on. You cannot fight your disease effectively unless you know as much as there is to know about it.

Don't just lie back and let your doctors 'do' things to you. Insist on sharing in the care of your body. Insist on being consulted. Get out of bed if you want to get out of bed and your doctors cannot give you any solid reasons why you should stay there.

3. Learn to respect yourself too. Build up your self-confidence and your confidence in your abilities.

Imagine that you are a copywriter for an advertising agency and prepare a campaign designed to sell yourself to the world. People who develop – and die of – cancer often have a low opinion of themselves. Build up your confidence and you'll not only suffer less pain, but you'll also live longer too. Remember that every year many thousands of patients defeat cancer completely.

4. The TENS device has been shown to be extremely effective as a pain reliever for cancer patients. And unlike many of the powerful drugs that are used to combat cancer pain, it does not produce any unpleasant or uncomfortable side effects.

Childbirth

As I've pointed out several times in this book, it really isn't possible to compare different types of pain in any genuinely objective way. The pains of childbirth, however, are reckoned by a good many experts to be among the worst of all pains.

Why then do so many women keep having babies? And why do they make so remarkably little fuss about it? After all, there is plenty of evidence to show that women tend to have a lower pain tolerance than men.

There are two probable explanations.

First, for most women having a baby is a joyful occasion. Like soldiers in a battle, their pains are endured in a worthwhile cause. Their minds are occupied with their new baby and not with their pain. To support this theory there is evidence available showing that women suffer far more pain if they have a baby that they don't really want.

Second, our memory for pain is extremely poor. When we have a bad pain we think it is the end of the world. We think we're going to die. And we make all sorts of rash promises to ourselves and to our Maker. But when the pain has gone we forget all about our fears and our promises. Within a matter of months the woman who has sworn never to have another baby starts getting broody again.

The initial and main pains of childbirth are produced when the powerful muscles of the uterus start contracting. These rhythmic contractions are designed to pull on the cervix or neck of the womb until it begins to open up. Once the cervix has expanded enough for the baby's head to get through, then the muscles of the uterus keep contracting in order to push both the baby and the placenta through the cervix and into the vagina.

Childbirth pains are felt in two main areas. Because the uterus gets its nerve supply from the middle level of the spinal cord the initial cramping contraction pains are felt in the middle of the back, at about waist level. And because the muscles and tissues of the vagina have to be stretched fairly considerably there will be some pain there too. If a woman is having her first baby, and her vaginal tissues have to be stretched for the first time, then obviously the pain she feels here is considerably worse than if she has had a number of babies before. The pain produced by the contracting muscles of the uterus may continue for a day or two after the baby has been born and if the skin around the vagina has been torn or cut then there may be additional pain there too.

Pain Control Programme in practice

Many of the elements of my Pain Control Programme may relieve the pains of childbirth. For example:

1. Fear and anxiety about what is happening commonly makes the pains of childbirth far worse than they need be. If you are about to have a baby you should spend some time reading about what happens during childbirth. Where possible you should also try to establish some sort of rapport with the doctor or midwife who will deliver your baby.

2. Women who learn how to relax their minds and their bodies suffer far less from pain during childbirth. Different experts recommend different types of relaxation exercise, but the relaxation methods described on pages 80ff. and 145ff. will work just as well for the pains of childbirth as with any other pain.

It is, I think, important to point out that women who learn to relax properly will not necessarily be able to banish all pain during childbirth. They may still need help from their doctors, and should not feel guilty if they need to ask for help. But the important point to remember is that women who learn how to relax properly will need far fewer pain killers than women who don't learn how to relax.

3. Warm baths will often help relieve the pains which persist after childbirth. To help prevent infection developing, a little salt can be added to the bath water.

4. Women who are approaching childbirth should try to spend as much time as possible concentrating on the baby they are about to have rather than on the pains they may suffer. By replacing unpleasant expectations about pain with happy thoughts of the baby she is about to have a mother can often minimize the amount of pain-killing relief she requires.

5. Constipation will make childbirth pains far worse. By eating high-fibre foods and plenty of fresh fruit it is possible to avoid constipation and therefore minimize pain during and after childbirth.

6. If you are planning a pregnancy, increase the power and strength of the muscles in your pelvic area. Since the muscles that control your vaginal walls also control the flow of urine from your bladder it is not difficult to learn how to do this. Sit on the lavatory with your legs apart and your arms resting on your thighs. You should then force a little urine out and almost immediately use the muscles between the tops of your thighs to stop the flow. For the next few minutes you should continue to pass teaspoonfuls of urine in bursts, contracting your muscles to control the flow. After practising like this for a while you will be able to contract and relax the relevant muscles without needing to pass urine. And then you will be able to practise the exercise whatever else you are doing and wherever you are: at home or at work.

Remember that the stronger your muscles are, the less pain you're likely to suffer during or after childbirth.

Headaches

Headaches are so common that four out of every five people get them. They can be caused by all sorts of things. You can get a headache if you strain your eyes, drink too much alcohol, have bad teeth, eat ice cream or develop arthritis in your neck. Some people even get headaches every time they have an orgasm. Very, very occasionally a headache may be caused by a brain tumour. (This is the diagnosis most people worry about when they get a headache. The truth is that brain tumours are extremely rare. One expert recently surveyed 1,152 patients who had been referred to a hospital specialist because their general practitioners thought that they might have brain tumours. In fact only one of that selected group of headache sufferers actually had a brain tumour.)

The great majority of headaches aren't caused by any of these problems. They are caused by stress, fear, anxiety and tension. Something like 98 per cent of all headaches – and that includes the types of headache known as 'tension headaches' and 'migraines' – fall into this category.

Sadly, despite the fact that the headache is probably the commonest single medical symptom requiring treatment or advice, headache sufferers usually do not get very much satisfaction from their doctors. When consulted by headache sufferers most doctors respond by reaching for their prescription pads and writing out a prescription either for a mild aspirin-like pain killer or for a tranquilliser. The fact is, however, that neither of these two drug types is particularly useful. Pain killers do nothing other than cover up the symptoms, and prescribing a pain killer for a headache is rather like offering a gallon of petrol to a motorist who has got a hole in his petrol tank. Tranquillizers are, if anything, less appropriate. That's the depressing news.

The cheering news is that the majority of headache sufferers can learn how to deal with their problem themselves by studying my Pain Control Programme.

Pain Control Programme in practice

Any or all of the elements of my Pain Control Programme may relieve headaches. For example:

1. If you are a regular headache sufferer you must try and find out whether there is anything in particular causing your headache. Keep a record of the times when your headaches start, how long they last, what other symptoms you develop and what treatments you find most effective. If you keep a full record like this then you may spot a pattern. Perhaps you only get headaches when you've eaten Chinese food (the 'Chinese Food Syndrome' has been shown to be caused by monosodium glutamate, which is widely used in Chinese cooking). Or maybe your headaches only develop when you've been smoking (tobacco can produce migraine headaches).

It is well worth remembering that many common foodstuffs may be responsible for headaches. Sugar, wheat, citrus fruits such as oranges and lemons, chocolate, cheese and milk are among the most commonly responsible foodstuffs. If you suspect that your headache could be caused by any specific foodstuff, it will obviously be sensible to cut out that particular food.

Remember that although we generally regard caffeine as a harmful mild stimulant it is in fact a powerful and extremely addictive drug which can cause headaches in several different ways. It can exacerbate stress and tension. If you are an addict, going without a 'fix' can result in a withdrawal headache. If you are a regular tea or coffee drinker (coffee contains slightly more caffeine than tea and ground coffee contains more caffeine than instant coffee) and you feel uncomfortable if you go too long without a cup of your favourite beverage, your headaches may well be a result of your caffeine consumption. Try avoiding coffee, tea, cola drinks and chocolate completely for a week. If your headaches are becoming less frequent by then, then you may have found the answer.

It isn't just eating the wrong sorts of food that can cause headaches, however. If you regularly miss meals then you may get headaches caused by the development of a low blood sugar level. This is particularly likely if your headaches are invariably worst when you get up first thing in the morning. If this is the case then try having a snack later in the evening – it may be all you need to keep your blood sugar levels up a little higher.

The other fairly common cause of headaches is eyestrain. If you get headaches after studying or reading all day then you should remember that the majority of headaches resulting from close work are caused by poor lighting. Anyone reading for long periods of time should have an adjustable reading lamp directed straight on to the area of work and a good, overhead general light too. When reading a book or studying texts the papers which are being used should stand at an angle of about 45 degrees to the desk. Most good stationers sell book rests and stands, which are well worth buying. They cost far less that a lifetime's supply of aspirin tablets.

2. By far the commonest cause of headaches developing is stress and tension. Learning to relax mentally is an excellent way to deal with headaches that have already developed. It is also an excellent way of preventing headaches from developing.

I suggest that you read through the section starting on page 80 and then try one or more of the dream sequences that I have described or invent one of your own. Lie down, make yourself comfortable and imagine that you can hear the sound of the birds singing or the sound of the waves breaking on the shore.

Do please remember that if you want to use this technique for dealing with a headache you must practise it when you are well.

3. When a headache is caused by muscle tension you'll benefit if you can relax the muscles of your head and neck. If you deliberately clench the muscles of your left fist then you'll feel the muscles go tight and uncomfortable. A pain will eventually develop in your fist. Much the same sort of thing can happen in your head when you are under pressure. The muscles of your neck, face, head and scalp all become tight. Your eyes will be screwed up and your muscle tension will eventually lead to a headache. You can get rid of that sort of tension by deliberately relaxing the muscles involved. Try to feel the muscles become free and loose, and your pains will gradually disappear.

4. We often use headaches as an excuse for not doing something that we don't want to do. A man will develop a 'headache' in order to avoid having to attend a dance he doesn't want to go too. A woman will develop a 'headache' as an excuse to avoid sex.

If you use the headache excuse often enough then eventually your body will begin to 'give' you headaches on other occasions to. As far as your mind is concerned the headache will become a universal solution to problems that seem to have no answer. Your mind will learn to create a headache when it doesn't know how to cope. If you suspect that you may be using your headaches as an excuse to avoid doing things, then try to identify – and deal with – the problems which lie behind the excuses.

5. Many people who regularly suffer from headaches do so because they are constantly being manipulated into doing things that they really don't want to do. By asserting yourself, standing up for yourself and gaining more confidence in yourself and your own decisions then you may well be able to stop yourself getting headaches. See page 107 for advice on how to assert yourself.

6. Migraine headaches seem to be getting more and more common these days. Apart from a one-sided headache the main symptoms usually include a mood change, itchy eyes, a stuffed-up nose, nausea and an increased sensitivity to

light and noise. Most sufferers start getting migraines before they reach the age of twenty, and three times as many women as men get migraines.

There is still some confusion about precisely what happens during a migraine attack, but it seems that the problem is largely a result of the body's inappropriate response to stress. Misled into thinking that it can cope with a stressful situation by preparing muscles for direct physical action, the body increases the supply of blood to the muscles and reduces the supply to the brain. Then, when the threat seems to be lifting, the blood vessels to the brain reopen and the blood surges into the tissues. It is this sudden flow of blood which seems to cause the pain associated with a migraine attack.

Doctors have proved quite incapable of dealing with most migraine attacks. But many sufferers have benefited enormously by using imagery techniques. Since the pain associated with a migraine attack is caused primarily by the constriction of the blood vessels supplying the brain, the aim of any imagery procedure must be to help enlarge the vessels concerned. The trouble is, of course, that it is extremely difficult to open up the arteries supplying the brain – largely because it is difficult to tell just how effective an imagery exercise is since neither the vessels nor the brain can be seen.

However, since the blood vessels to the hands are constricted whenever the blood vessels to the brain are constricted there is a solution: at the very first sign of a migraine developing (and most patients get some warning sign) you must make a conscious effort to direct blood into your hands.

This is easier than it sounds. You simply need to imagine that your hands are getting warmer and warmer. As you do this your blood vessels will open up to ensure that more blood flows into the tissues. And as the blood vessels in your hands open up, so the blood vessels to your brain will open up too. Trials have shown that 80 per cent of migraine sufferers can help themselves in this way.

Incidentally, it has been shown that the blood vessels which supply the heart can also be enlarged in exactly the same way, and this technique has also been successfully used to overcome the anginal pains of early heart disease.

7. Neck, head and shoulder massage is an excellent way to get rid of tension headaches. If you can find a willing friend get him (or her) to stand behind you while you are sitting down, and to massage the muscles at the back of your neck and in your shoulders. Get him to massage your scalp too. If you can't find a willing friend then you can try massaging yourself (see page 119 for more details).

8. TENS devices and ice packs are both useful for controlling headaches. There is more information about these two techniques on pages 120 and 131.

Period Pains

.Something like 50 per cent of all women who menstruate get period pains that are more than just mildly troublesome. Many get pains which are so bad that they are incapacitating.

Period pains are usually divided into two main groups: those which start at or around puberty (known as primary dysmenorrhoea) and those which start after years of painless or relatively painless menstruation (known as secondary dysmenorrhoea).

The onset of pain in primary dysmenorrhoea is usually at puberty and it is thought to be caused by uterine contractions induced by the local production of prostaglandins. These substances are of a similar type to the one that is produced during childbirth, and the period pains that it produces are similar to the pains associated with childbirth. The pain is usually colicky, starting a few hours before menstruation and lasting for about a day; it is sometimes accompanied by nausea, sweating, fainting and constipation. The pain is usually situated in the lower part of the abdomen, and often goes down into the buttocks and thighs too.

Two-thirds of the girls who develop primary dysmenorrhoea have a family history of such pains, and many girls who suffer badly have been warned at considerable length (usually by their mothers) to expect a lot of pain and suffering when their periods start. At the very least most girls who suffer from primary dysmenorrhoea will have usually seen their mothers suffering from pain, and will have therefore learnt to associate menstrual periods with considerable amounts of pain and suffering.

Secondary dysmenorrhoea can be produced in a number of different ways. By definition it always develops after years of pain-free menstruation and can be caused by infections, endometriosis, pelvic inflammatory disease, polyps, cancer, fibroids, bowel disorders, urinary problems, skeletal disorders, intra-uterine contraceptive devices and just about anything else you can think of too – including anxiety and tension, of course.

Most doctors still treat period pains with pills, and there are many pills available without a prescription. Yet there is a great deal of evidence now available to show that mental attitudes play an important part in the development of period pains. And there is evidence to show that even where relaxation or imagery techniques do not work, period pains can often be conquered by using techniques such as electrical stimulation and the application of heat.

Pain Control Programme in practice

Any or all of the elements of my Pain Control Programme may be used in the treatment of period pains. For example:

1. Imagery is an excellent way of dealing with the abdominal pains associated with menstruation. There are two specific techniques that are well worth trying.

First, imagine that your right hand is as cold as it can possibly be. Try to freeze it so much that it feels quite numb. Then place your frozen hand over the area where your abdominal pain is greatest and let the numbness soak down through your abdominal wall to the site where it is needed most.

Second, try clasping your right hand as tightly as you possibly can, imagining in your mind that, as the muscles of your hand contract so the muscles of your uterus contract too. Try to see your hand as your uterus or womb. Keep your hand like this for a minute or two. Now, slowly relax the muscles of your hand and allow your fingers to unfold. As you do this your uterine muscles will relax too and your pain will slowly fade away.

2. Many of the pains associated with menstruation are

caused by fear and embarrassment and even shame. (The common and descriptive word 'curse' which is often used to describe menstruation goes back to the days when women who were menstruating were thought to be accursed in some way and were kept in huts well away from their village.) A young girl who understands what is happening when she menstruates is far less likely to suffer from pain than a young girl who has no idea about what is happening to her.

3. Mental relaxation can prove extremely beneficial. Any of the techniques described on pages 80ff. can be tried, although you will obviously benefit more if you create your own dream sequences and learn to use them whenever your period pain is developing.

4. Heat and warmth can help alleviate period pains very effectively. A warm bath may help, but a hot-water bottle (carefully wrapped in a thin towel to prevent burning) is probably the most effective way of applying heat to the lower abdomen.

5. If you suffer from severe and persistent period pains then you should perhaps invest in a TENS device. As I have explained elsewhere, the main advantage of the TENS device is that it uses your body's own pain-suppressing mechanisms, and can therefore have no harmful effects.

Index